HIPAA FOR HEALTH CARE PROFESSIONALS

DAN KRAGER

CAROLE KRAGER, C.C.A.

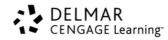

DELMAR
CENGAGE Learning

Australia • Brazil • Japan • Korea • Mexico • Singapore • Spain • United Kingdom • United States

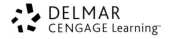

HIPAA for Health Care Professionals
Dan Krager and Carole Krager

Vice President, Career and
Professional Editorial:
Dave Garza

Director of Learning Solutions:
Matthew Kane

Managing Editor:
Marah Bellegarde

Acquisitions Editor:
Matthew Seeley

Editorial Assistant:
Megan Tarquinio

Vice President, Career and
Professional Marketing:
Jennifer McAvey

Marketing Manager:
Michele McTighe

Marketing Coordinator:
Chelsey Iaquinta

Production Director:
Carolyn Miller

Production Manager:
Andrew Crouth

Content Project Manager:
Katie Wachtl

Senior Art Director:
Jack Pendleton

Technology Project Manager:
Christopher Catalina

Production Technology Analyst:
Thomas Stover

For product information and technology assistance, contact us at
Cengage Learning Customer & Sales Support, 1-800-354-9706

For permission to use material from this text or product, submit all requests online at **cengage.com/permissions**

Further permissions questions can be emailed to
permissionrequest@cengage.com

Library of Congress Control Number: 2007943956

ISBN-13: 978-1-4180-8053-2

ISBN-10: 1-4180-8053-5

Delmar
Executive Woods
5 Maxwell Drive
Clifton Park, NY 12065-2919
USA

Cengage Learning products are represented in Canada by Nelson Education, Ltd.

For your course and learning solutions, visit **academic.cengage.com**

Purchase any of our products at your local college store or at our preferred online store **www.ichapters.com**

Notice to the Reader

Publisher does not warrant or guarantee any of the products described herein or perform any independent analysis in connection with any of the product information contained herein. Publisher does not assume, and expressly disclaims, any obligation to obtain and include information other than that provided to it by the manufacturer. The reader is expressly warned to consider and adopt all safety precautions that might be indicated by the activities described herein and to avoid all potential hazards. By following the instructions contained herein, the reader willingly assumes all risks in connection with such instructions. The publisher makes no representations or warranties of any kind, including but not limited to, the warranties of fitness for particular purpose or merchant ability, nor are any such representations implied with respect to the material set forth herein, and the publisher takes no responsibility with respect to such material. The publisher shall not be liable for any special, consequential, or exemplary damages resulting, in whole or part, from the reader's use of, or reliance upon, this material.

Printed in Canada
3 4 5 6 7 12 11 10 09

PREFACE

HIPAA for Health Care Professionals is a teaching/learning tool for both students and members of the health care workforce. HIPAA (Health Insurance Portability and Accountability Act) law mandates training of all new employees and retraining on a routine basis for every employee within health care. Training includes anyone who has possible contact with protected health information. Beginning in 2003, many people were concerned about what HIPAA would mean to the health care industry. Some of these concerns were valid, and many others were quite extreme. We hope to show the reasonableness of this law and how the health care industry can comply and more fully protect individual health information.

In teaching a course in medical insurance and coding, the author found HIPAA books that were written in haste. Most were technically accurate but did not cover all areas of HIPAA. Other more comprehensive texts were written with additions to include HIPAA law but were not suitable to explain the complete scope of the law. A basic understanding of how health care is delivered today will contribute to greater understanding. A solid text capable of stimulating in-depth learning is needed when a health care professional faces critical compliance decisions.

Methods of Research

Instead of taking opinions from here and there, the authors researched the government Web sites, the *Federal Register,* and actual advice published by the Department of Health and Human Services concerning how to understand the rules. Government wording can be quite confusing so care was taken to define concepts as the government defines them and carefully present the intent of the law in everyday language.

Organization

Care was taken to study one element of HIPAA at a time to ensure the reader's understanding. *HIPAA for Health Care Professionals* is written for easy reading. Knowledge of medical terminology is not required. Coverage includes an introduction to HIPAA concepts, explanation of privacy rule, transactions and code sets, security rules and their impact on the workplace, and a discussion of myths surrounding HIPAA. Forms and resources that can be used in the workplace are included in the appendix.

Features

Each chapter contains the following:

- *Chapter objectives* and a *key term list* to help the reader focus their learning

- *Think About It* features found at the beginning of each chapter as well as throughout the chapter stimulate reflection about concepts discussed. The questions posed can be discussed prior to reading and then addressed later to see if first impressions were correct.

- *True Stories* and *Scenarios* illustrate actual real-life happenings and emphasize the importance of HIPAA compliance.

- *Review Questions* found at the end of chapter allow the reader to check their understanding of chapter concepts.

Also available:

WebTutor on Web CT to Accompany HIPAA for Health Care Professionals
ISBN: 1418080551
WebTutor on Blackboard to Accompany HIPAA for Health Care Professionals
ISBN: 141808056X

Designed to complement the book, WebTutor is a Web-based teaching and learning aid that reinforces and clarifies complex concepts. This valuable resource includes key concepts, Web links, discussion questions, glossary, and additional quizzes. The Web CT and Blackboard platforms also provide rich communication tools to instructors and students, including a course calendar, chat, e-mail, and threaded discussions.

Instructor Resources

An *Electronic Classroom Manager* is available to instructors.
ISBN 1-4180-8054-3
Included in the package:

- *Instructor's Manual,* including answers to *Think About It* questions and *Review Questions,* and ideas on how material can be used in professional training scenarios

- 100 *PowerPoint slides* to assist in classroom presentations and lectures

- *Computerized Test Bank* containing 250 questions; allows users to generate tests with a few clicks of a button!

ABOUT THE AUTHORS

Dan Krager is Manager of Information Systems, Richland Memorial Hospital, Olney, IL; HIPAA Officer for Richland Memorial Hospital; HIPAA Security Officer for Richland Memorial Hospital; Bachelor of Science, Wheaton College, Wheaton, Illinois Certified Network Engineer in Novell Systems, Cisco systems, and Linux training; and has over 15 years experience in computer and network applications for hospital settings. As HIPAA Officer and HIPAA Security Officer, Dan enabled Richland Memorial Hospital to move toward compliance. He worked closely with the Illinois Hospital Association to build a statewide infrastructure that enables health care organizations to interconnect electronically.

Carole H. Krager is Instructor at Olney Central College campus of Illinois Eastern Community College, Olney, IL in the Business Department, teaching Medical Insurance and Coding; Bachelor of Science, Wheaton College, Wheaton, IL; experienced in clinic billing; trained in diagnosis coding at Triton College, River Grove, IL; experienced in outpatient hospital coding; member of the American Health Information Management Association and Certified Coding Assistant (CCA) proficiency. Carole has been an educator for more than 25 years and has successfully communicated in an easy-to-understand manner. She has been trained in teaching students who learn outside the norm. Experience with billing and coding enabled her to understand the inner workings of both physician and hospital offices.

ACKNOWLEDGEMENTS

We wish to thank members of Richland (IL) Memorial Hospital for their assistance. We have listened to how they moved to HIPAA compliance and found some pitfalls. We hope you will avoid those pitfalls through full understanding of the HIPAA rulings. The specific friends are Lezlie Lambird, Medical Records Department; Tom Stein, Pharmacy Department; Julie Struble, Admitting Department; Lana Royse, Quality Assurance Improvement; Randy Bishop, Diagnostic Imaging Department; Bruce Maxwell, Emergency Department; Jack Fleeharty, Ambulance Department; and Bob Gammon, Food Service Department.

We would like to send a special thank you to the reviewers of our manuscript. Their input was invaluable.

Christa Bartlett, CMA-CPC
Assistant Professor
University of Alaska Fairbanks/Tanana Valley Campus
Fairbanks, Alaska

Mark Forquer, BS, Ed, NCMA
Medical Assistant Instructor
Advanced Career Training
Jacksonville, Florida

Carolyn H. Greene, BS, MBA, RHE
Academic Dean, School of Health Sciences
Program Director Health Services Management
Virginia College at Birmingham
Birmingham, Alabama

Barbara Hogg, MLT, RN, BSN
Director of Distance Learning
South Arkansas Community College
El Dorado, Arizona

Stacey May, CST
Program Director/Instructor of Surgical Technology
and Surgical Assisting South Plains College
Lubbock, Texas

We have endeavored to thoroughly cover the areas of HIPAA that have brought the most misunderstanding. Certainly there are gray areas that health care professionals will encounter. If we can be of assistance to clarify and offer a carefully considered opinion, we certainly welcome the opportunity. Our e-mail address is dkrager@otbnet.com and our mailing address is 4730 N Wilder Road, Olney, IL 62450.

CONTENTS

CHAPTER 3

TRANSACTIONS AND CODE SETS 54

CHAPTER 4

SECURITY RULE EXPLAINED 82

CHAPTER 5

UNIQUE HEALTH IDENTIFIERS AND HIPAA MYTHS 109

APPENDIX

HIPAA FOR HEALTH CARE PROFESSIONALS 131

GLOSSARY 157

INDEX 166

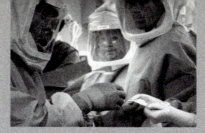

CHAPTER

1

INTRODUCTION TO HIPAA

OBJECTIVES

Understand reasons for the Health Insurance Portability and Accountability Act of 1996.

Recognize the scope of HIPAA law for both health care and the insurance industry.

Appreciate the need to protect the privacy and security of health information.

Describe the types of health care providers that are "covered entities."

Explain the importance of the HIPAA Officer.

Discuss the many areas in the delivery of health care that are affected by HIPAA through an imaginary scenario.

KEY TERMS

covered entity
Department of Health and Human Services (DHHS)
group health plan
health care clearinghouse
health care providers

Health Insurance Portability and Accountability Act of 1996 (HIPAA)
HIPAA officer
individually identifiable health information (IIHI)

need to know
privacy
protected health information (PHI)
security
transactions

INTRODUCTION

*I*n *the True Story account below, private information was shared inappropriately. Health information could have been easily used to restrict or terminate employment. Improperly disclosed health information could have been used in many ways that injured the reputation of another. It revealed information that allowed for misuse by those who had no business knowing specific health information about another person. These and other accounts accumulated and placed pressure on Congress to enact legislation to safeguard everyone's medical information. Since the mid-1970s, United States representatives and senators had proposed legislation to reform various elements of the health care industry. Most proposals failed, and a compromise was not reached until 1996 when the 104th Congress focused upon six issues.*

1. To improve portability and continuity in the group and individual insurance markets
2. To combat waste, fraud, and abuse in health insurance and health care delivery
3. To promote the use of medical savings accounts (MSAs)
4. To improve access to long-term care services and coverage
5. To simplify the administration of health insurance
6. To provide a means to pay for reforms, and other related purposes

The **Health Insurance Portability and Accountability Act of 1996 (HIPAA),** *now known as HIPAA, mandated many changes to health insurance carriers and health care providers. There are four main areas where the law has changed the way business is conducted in the health care industry.*

1. *Privacy* of health information
2. Standards for *electronic transactions* of health information and claims
3. *Security* of electronic health information
4. *National identifiers* for the parties in health care transactions

Privacy protection is the most talked-about ruling. These rules affect all health care providers, people, and organizations that have any access to health care records. We will cover each of these four areas with special emphasis on privacy and security issues.

Think About It

1. Give an example of what you have heard about the law called HIPAA.
2. Why does the HIPAA law stir up so much talk?
3. Debate the reasons for keeping health information private. What are reasons for disclosure? What are reasons for privacy? What are reasons for security?
4. Give examples of how people might be hurt when certain medical information is revealed to employers, family members, friends, and financial organizations.

True Story

An Atlanta truck driver lost his job in early 1998 after his employer learned from his insurance company that he had sought treatment for a drinking problem. (Appleby, 2000).

True Story

After suffering a work-related injury to her wrist, Roni Breite authorized her insurance company to release information pertaining to her wrist ailment to her employer. When she had the opportunity to review her medical records, the file contained her entire medical history, including records on recent fertility treatment and pregnancy loss. (McCarthy, 1999).

How the Rules Came into Existence

The Health Insurance Portability and Accountability Act of 1996 passed both houses of Congress and became Public Law 104-191. By signing this bill, President Clinton confirmed a process that generated new rules for health insurance plans and health care providers plus penalties for not complying. The final law was subdivided into seven titles.

Title I – Health Care Access, Portability, and Renewability

Title II – Preventing Health Care Fraud and Abuse; Administrative Simplification; Medical Liability Reform

Title III – Tax-related Health Provisions

Title IV – Application and Enforcement of Group Health Plan Requirements

Title V – Revenue Offsets

Title XI (11) – General Provisions, Peer Review, Administrative Simplification

Title XXVII (27) – Assuring Portability, Availability and Renewability of Health Insurance Coverage(H.R. 3103, 1996)

The inclusion of Title II—Administrative Simplification—affects practices and procedures of **health care providers**. A health care provider is anyone or organization that furnishes, bills, or is paid for health care in the normal course of business. Congress left the details to the secretary of the **Department of Health and Human Services (DHHS)** to develop rulings in accordance to the Public Law 104-191, or HIPAA. Since the DHHS rulings are not legislative law, the DHHS can adjust, amend, delete, or change the rulings at any time. Modifications to the first rulings are already being issued.

In October 1997, Congress passed a clarification of HIPAA. This simplified the administration of medical billing procedures because all **transactions** were to be transmitted electronically using the industry-wide standards of electronic data interchange (EDI). "Providers are given the option of whether to conduct the transactions electronically or 'on paper,' but if they elect to conduct them electronically, they must use the standards agreed upon through the law." The goal is to *"simplify the administration of the nation's health care system and improve its efficiency and effectiveness."* Payers are required to accept these transmissions and are not to delay a transaction, or adversely affect the provider who conducts transactions electronically" (Hobson, 1997). All health care providers, health plans, and health care clearinghouses that transmit protected health information electronically are treated equally regarding payment for health care. Failure for noncompliance is clearly outlined. The DHHS wrote rulings so that all parties, large and small, could comply with a nationwide standard. Small private insurance providers and government agencies are to be treated equally, and they must treat each health care provider the same. The flow of information and reimbursements becomes more efficient. This results in savings in the cost of insurance and providing health care.

The secretary of the DHHS approved final rules and released the rules in the *Federal Register* and to the public. April 2003 was selected for the beginning of enforcement. All parties were required to comply 24 months after the effective date. Once a ruling has been adopted, it is in force for a period of at least 12 months. After that time it may be amended or changed. All parties affected by HIPAA are required to keep up to date with any changes. That responsibility lies with each organization under HIPAA law.

TITLES OF HIPAA LAW

The main focus of the law is to provide a means for people to carry insurance coverage from one health insurance company to another *and* to simplify communication between health insurance plans and health care providers. Here is a short overview of the major portions.

Title I: Health Insurance Access, Portability, and Renewal

Title I (1): Health Care Access Portability and Renewability increases the portability of health insurance. It changes the rules concerning preexisting condition exclusions. When a worker changes jobs or is released from work, that worker can continue health coverage even with a preexisting condition. This law prohibits health insurance coverage discrimination based on health status. It also guarantees renewability for certain group health plans.

Title II: Preventing Health Care Fraud and Abuse; Administrative Simplification; Medical Liability Reform

Title II (2): Preventing Health Care Fraud and Abuse; Administrative Simplification; Medical Liability Reform is the portion of the bill that speaks to the health provider and how they interact with the insurance network.

The important areas of concern are the following:

1. Prevent fraud and abuse in delivering and paying for health care.

2. Improve the Medicare program and other programs through efficient and effective standards.

3. Establish standards for all electronic transmission of certain health information. (H.R. 3103, 1996).

Title II established a fraud and abuse control program and a method of collecting health information. It spelled out civil and criminal penalties for guilty parties when either abuse or fraud events are documented. Each state had enacted regulations governing the health insurance companies within their jurisdiction. Each state had regulations concerning abuse. Only federal programs, such as Medicare, Medicaid, TRICARE, and the Civilian Health and Medical Program of the Veterans Administration (CHAMPVA) had federal authority to prosecute situations of fraud. All covered entities must comply with federal law as a minimum no matter where they are located. Only when state or local laws are more stringent will the state or local law be held as the standard for the providers in that particular area.

The *Administrative Simplification* portion of HIPAA is where **privacy** and **security** issues relating to **protected health information (PHI)** are explained. The Privacy Rule and Security Rule have unique perspectives and yet overlap significantly. Health care providers, health plans, and health care clearinghouses that hold or transmit PHI in any form or media whether electronic, paper, or oral must comply with the Privacy Rule. The *Privacy Rule* states how PHI is to be handled. It explains when and to whom PHI may be shared, states when authorization is necessary, and requires policies that protect disclosure of information that is in any form: electronic, paper, video, recordings, film, or other.

The *Security Rule* speaks to the protection of electronic PHI (e-PHI). Any health care provider, health plan, and health care clearinghouse that transmits or receives PHI *electronically* must comply with the Administrative Simplification portion also. Any health information that is sent via electronic means, not printed on paper, must be kept secure from intrusion, loss, and inappropriate disclosure. Separate but connected rulings are the Transaction and Code Set Rule (TCS) plus the Unique Identifier rulings that explain details of entity identifiers in a claims transaction. The *Transaction and Code Set Rule* details the form and elements to be used by all covered entities transmitting of e-PHI in relation to reimbursement.

The last portions of the Unique Identifier rulings are to be developed. These deal with the change to electronic media and how each entity in a standard transaction is identified on electronic health claims with unique *national identifiers*. This monumental task is partially finished with generating unique identification numbers for four groups.

1.   Health care providers—individuals and organizations

2.   Health plans or payers

3.   Health care clearinghouses

4.   Patients

With electronic media, there must be many safeguards built into electronic systems. Protection is needed from accidental disaster, unauthorized access, disclosure of only **"need to know"** information, and incidental disclosure to persons other than the patient or their representative. There were prior local laws and state statutes protecting health information that was in paper form. The Privacy and Security Rules have defined protections for nationwide uniformity. The Information Technology Department usually has the main responsibility to ensure compliance with the many facets of security.

Title IV: Group Health Plan Requirements

Title IV (4): Application and Enforcement of Group Health Plan Requirements amends the Consolidated Omnibus Budget Reconciliation Act of 1985 (COBRA). It details how group health plans must allow for portability, access, and renewability for members of a group health plan. A **group health plan** is defined as an employee welfare benefit plan that provides health coverage in the form of medical care and services through insurance, reimbursement, or other means for a group of employees and dependents. Many employers have arrangements for employees to participate in a health plan that includes any person employed by the organization—thus the group health plan. As workers move from one job to another, this law allows people the option to carry the same health insurance coverage to their new work situation instead of having to start over again with waiting periods for preexisting conditions or other similar conditions of coverage.

Other Titles in HIPAA

Title III (3): Tax-Related Health Provisions speaks about medical savings accounts (MSAs) and how employers handle these funds for employees, increasing the deduction for health insurance for self-employed individuals, long-term care insurance benefits, related consumer protection provisions, and income tax refund payments in relation to organ and tissue donations. A medical savings account is a tax-sheltered savings account similar to an individual retirement account (IRA), but earmarked for medical expenses only. Participating individuals can deposit money into this type of account and withdraw the funds throughout the year for medical expenses only. Deposits are 100 percent tax deductible for the self-employed and can be withdrawn by check or debit card to pay routine medical bills with tax-free dollars.

Title V (5): Revenue Offsets explains how the ruling changed the Internal Revenue Code of 1986 to generate more revenue to offset the HIPAA required costs. The other titles in the bill cover minor issues and are short in length. They clarify certain items of the law.

PHI is defined by the Centers for Medicare and Medicaid Services as **individually identifiable health information (IIHI)** transmitted or maintained in any form or medium, which is held by a covered entity or its business associate, and that

1. Identifies the individual or offers a reasonable basis for identification.

2. Is created or received by a covered entity or an employer.

3. Relates to a past, present, or future physical or mental condition; provision of health care; or payment for health care.

In short, PHI is the association of identifiers with diagnoses. The concern for privacy and security of PHI is now a very important part of the health care process from the federal level.

HIPAA: An Organizational and Business Challenge

All health care providers, health insurance plans, health care clearinghouses, payers of medical insurance, and other associated businesses have to adjust their practices to be in line with the HIPAA law. (Figure 1-1.) A **health care clearinghouse** is a business that submits health claims on behalf of a provider. Their function is to screen the claim for accuracy and be the intermediary between the health care provider and the insurance carrier. The Administrative Simplification portion of HIPAA has caused many

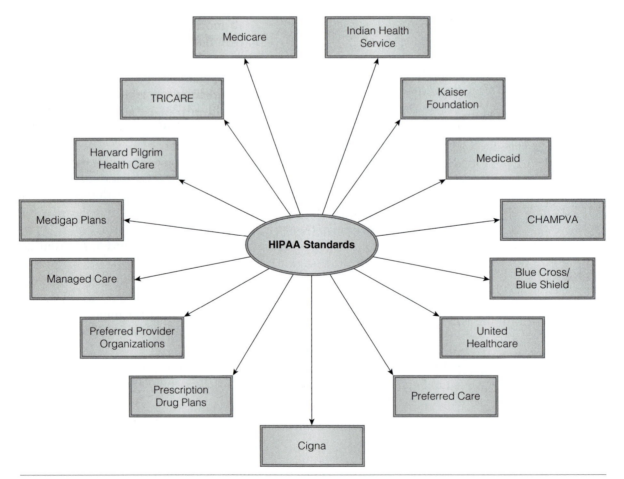

FIGURE 1-1 HIPPA applies to a wide variety of health care plans and providers.

changes within physician offices, clinics, hospitals, and outpatient offices as well as the insurance companies and ancillary providers of health services.

In 2003, the Centers for Medicare and Medicaid Services (CMS) verified that there were over 400 different ways to submit a health insurance claim. Only a federal law could compel all 50 states to comply with one standard. Many health insurance companies have headquarters that serve several states. Each state had standards unique to itself. Health insurance carriers could also demand certain forms or styles of claims submission. This federal ruling requires one standard form for submission of health claims thus eliminated customizing claims. The title of "Administrative Simplification" describes a major intent of this ruling. Business office personnel can submit one form electronically with confidence that as long as codes and patient data are accurate, the claim will be paid in a timely manner.

Health care providers are not yet required by HIPAA to conduct all transactions electronically. Further details concerning exceptions are listed in Chapter three, "Transactions and Code Sets." However, if health care providers transmit even one claim electronically, they will need to comply with the HIPAA standardized electronic format. Private insurance companies are also encouraged in this direction because the electronic process has the potential for significant savings. Greater efficiency is the result of this change. The supply of paper, the sorting of paper, the storage and final long-term archival storage of paper is currently a large cost of doing business. A study shows that it takes at least seven people to manage one single piece of paper. Few providers have considered a disaster plan to protect or replace lost paper records. With electronic data and transmissions, the need for paper, the accompanying file cabinets, and the space to house the cabinets is a thing of the past.

Seven People Manage One Piece of Paper

1. Someone fills it with data.

2. Someone authenticates it.

3. Someone has to distribute it.

4. Someone converts the data to meaningful information (reads it or makes a report).

5. Someone has to file it.

6. Someone has to retrieve it.

7. Someone has to manage the final disposition of it, whether it is stored or destroyed.

Who Is a "Covered Entity?"

The term "**covered entity**" is part of the HIPAA language. There are three categories of covered entities in the HIPAA law. The first is any health plan. This is a company, individual, or group that agrees to pay part or all of the medical care for the people included in their coverage. There are many types of health plans—dental plans, vision plans, and prescription drug insurers—besides the more traditional health insurance plans. Health plans include health maintenance organizations, Medicare, Medicaid, Medicare Plus Choice, Medicare supplemental insurers, Indian health service programs, veterans health care program (CHAMPVA), and the Civilian Health and Medical Program of the Uniformed Services, now called TRICARE. As of 2003, the Medicare Prescription Drug, Improvement, and Modernization Act authorized prescription drug card sponsors to act as covered entities. These sponsors are a subset of the health plan definition of covered entity. A prescription drug card sponsor is a non-governmental entity that is certified under federal law to offer a prescription drug plan (PDP), contract, or policy. This defines a prescription drug plan (PDP) as a covered entity since it receives e-PHI in order to determine reimbursement.

An exception to the designation of covered entity is given to an employer who has less than 50 employees *and* is "self-insured" (pays for medical costs from their own funds within the company). Insurance companies who provide health coverage are covered entities under HIPAA law. Insurance companies are referred to as third-party payers.

Certain Insurance Payers Are Not Covered Entities

Note: Not all insurance payers are covered entities. Insurance underwriters such as automobile, property, life, casualty, and workers compensation are not health plans and do not come under this category. These types of insurance carriers are not defined as covered entities, yet they do have access to PHI in order to process claims. It is important to understand this distinction when transmitting e-PHI. Only the minimum necessary information is to be shared with noncovered entities.

The second type of covered entity is a health care provider, a provider of medical or other health services and any other person who furnishes, bills, or is paid for health care in the normal course of business. Health care has a broad definition. It covers care, services, or supplies related to the health of an individual. It includes, but is not limited to, the following:

1. Preventative, diagnostic, rehabilitative, maintenance, or palliative care, and counseling, service, assessment, or procedure with respect

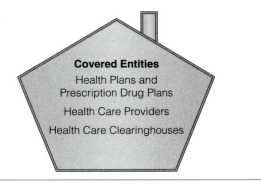

Covered Entities

Health Plans and
Prescription Drug Plans

Health Care Providers

Health Care Clearinghouses

FIGURE 1-2   Only these three types of organizations are responsible to the federal government to be in compliance with HIPAA regulations.

to the physical or mental condition, or functional status, of an individual or that affect the structure or function of the body.

2. Sale or dispensing of a drug, device, equipment, or other item in accordance with a prescription. (Covered Entity Chart, 2005).

Some atypical providers of health care are taxicab companies, carpenters, and home help personnel. These are generally exempt from the definition of covered entity. However, steps are being taken to move these atypical providers into a standardized electronic process in order to provide payment for their services. (Are You a Covered Entity … and When Does Rule 1 Apply?, 2001). See Appendix A for Covered Entity Charts from the CMS Web site to assist determination of who is a covered entity.

The third type of covered entity is a health care clearinghouse. This is a company that processes information it receives from health care providers and sends that information as an insurance claim for payment. Hospitals and small physician offices may defer the billing task to someone else whose business it is to keep abreast of changing rules. Clearinghouses handle claims from many providers and submit them in batches for processing. This allows the provider's office staff to concentrate on ensuring that claim information is as accurate as possible. The health care provider pays a fee to the clearinghouse to send and receive insurance information for him. The clearinghouse sends the health care provider credits from insurance payments minus their charge for the service. These clearinghouses are considered covered entities. See Figure 1-2 for a diagram of covered entities.

The HIPAA Officer

One person in each covered entity must be the designated **HIPAA officer** who coordinates and oversees the various aspects of compliance. Each covered entity should have a group of people, depending on the size of the organization, with responsibilities to oversee various segments of HIPAA compliance. (HIPAA Readiness Checklist, 2003). These segments may include a representative from

- Health information Management Department (Medical Records)
- Medical staff
- Information technology
- Legal advisory
- Patient accounts (business office)
- Risk management
- Satellite clinics
- Ancillary departments, such as social workers and chaplains

The HIPAA officer should have an understanding of the scope of the ruling and how each department will be affected. As time goes on, this officer must learn of any changes implemented to the ruling. The officer's responsibility includes yearly training and updating all staff members on current HIPAA mandates.

Depending on the size of the organization, there may be several officers. One person must be designated security officer to safeguard the security of the clinical records of patients. The HIPAA officer may also serve in this capacity. A privacy officer may be designated also. This person is to keep track of who has access to PHI. In a small office where one person may have many responsibilities, the functions of the various officers may be fulfilled by as few as two people, using one for backup.

SUMMARY

In 1996 Congress passed HIPAA. This law began a series of events reforming how health care insurance was managed by the insurance industry. The law provided that rulings written by the DHHS standardize the electronic processing of claims. These rulings simplified how health insurance claims are prepared and sent for payment. Insurance companies must provide individuals greater access to health care insurance when they change employers. They must also extend the coverage individuals need to new insurance carriers.

Four important issues were addressed that change the way health care providers interact with their patients and insurance carriers in the law.

- Protect the *privacy* of health information
- Standards for *electronic transactions* of health information and claims

- *Security* of electronic health information
- *National identifiers* for the parties in health care transactions

Congress stressed that the goal of HIPAA is to simplify the insurance claim process and provide faster payments for services rendered by the health care provider. However, while these changes are being implemented, many questions arise. Using explanations of this ruling and interpretations of the changes, one can understand the flow of PHI through the medical health care facility and physician's office and the measures mandated to protect it from unauthorized disclosures.

All branches of the health care industry are affected by HIPAA rulings. The scenario at the end of the chapter shows some of the extent to which staff members must understand how their actions are affected by the rulings.

The parties defined by HIPAA as "covered entities" include any health care provider, any health care clearinghouse, and any health insurance payer. An additional entity was defined in 2005—Medicare prescription drug card sponsors.

Each provider of health care must have an appointed HIPAA officer. This person, or persons for a large organization, is responsible to oversee that the facility is in compliance and there is proper documentation if governmental agents stop in.

❧ SCENARIO ❧

Where HIPAA Intersects Health Care

Let us consider a person needing health care. Read through the following scenario and see just how many places at which the ruling affects the delivery of health care. There are many concepts introduced that are specific to HIPAA. These will be addressed in more detail in later chapters. The reader might also consult the glossary at end of the book. This scenario will give an overview of the types of organizations and people who need to be fully aware of HIPAA regulations. This scenario does not try to include all of the health care settings that are touched by HIPAA, but the following includes many of them. HIPAA concepts are bolded.

Departments affected by HIPAA in scenario:

Ambulance services	Consulting physicians
Anesthesiologists	Dietary department
Auxiliary and volunteer workers	Emergency department
Certified nursing assistants (CNAs)	Health care clearinghouse firm
Clinical laboratory	Hospital information desk

(*continues*)

(continued)

Housekeeping	Reference Laboratory
Information Services/Technology	Registration
Licensed practical nurses (LPNs)	Research organizations
Medical staff	Surgical teams, including critical care and intensive care services
Medical Records Department	
Nursing staff	Switchboard operator
Operating room staff	Therapy Departments—Occupational, Speech, Rehabilitation
Outside laboratory	
Patient Accounts/Business Office	Transcriptionists
Pharmacy	Organizations outside health care:
Physician's office billing specialist	Law enforcement officials
Physician's receptionist	Repairmen working at a health care office
Psychiatry	Visiting clergy
Radiology	

HIPAA concepts identified in scenario:

access to psychotherapy notes	encrypted
audit trail	health care operations
authenticated	hospital directory
authorization requirements	individually identifiable health information (IIHI)
business associate	identifier standards
business as usual	minimum necessary
cases of victims of abuse, neglect, or domestic violence	need to know
	nonrepudiation security
covered entity	normal operations
data backup and disaster recovery plan	Notice of Privacy Practices
de-identified	"opt-out" of future requests or facility directory
designated ANSI X12 standard format	
designated code sets	personal representatives
designated record set	policy
disclosure of protected health information	precedence
electronic protected health information (e-PHI)	Privacy Rule

protected health information (PHI).

standardized transmission request and reply

purposes of treatment, payment
or health care operation (TPO)

treatment, payment, and health care
operations

reasonable

training

release of directory information

unauthorized access

request to amendment

victim(s) of abuse, neglect, or domestic
violence

research study

Security Rule

written accounting of disclosures

1) The mayor's elderly mother, Mrs. Elsa Goodman, is found unconscious in her home by a neighbor. The neighbor calls for an ambulance. Ambulance personnel find Mrs. Goodman on the floor of her home. They begin taking vitals and assessing her condition. The neighbor explains they often come to visit and forced the door open when they did not receive a response from Mrs. Goodman. The ambulance service personnel take a report from the neighbor and note that there is the possibility of elderly neglect. The ambulance staff transports Mrs. Goodman to the hospital.

   a) *Ambulance personnel may request information from people at the scene but are not to disclose any **protected health information** obtained from treating the patient.*

2) At the hospital, ambulance staff meets a longtime friend at doorway. The friend asks the ambulance member for more information about the patient. The ambulance staff just continues with his responsibility to care for the patient.

   a) *Disclosure of **protected health information** may be given only for **treatment, payment and normal health care operations**. The ambulance personnel may not comment on information they receive.*

3) Dr. Eveready, the Emergency Department doctor on duty, begins evaluation and finds a broken arm, badly bruised chest, and other bruises on Mrs. Goodman's body. The registration clerk begins to enter patient information into the hospital system.

   a) *The registration clerk needs to be trained in privacy and security matters. The hospital must document this **training**.*

   b) *The system should maintain an **audit trail** of information viewed and modified, showing who did it and when.*

   c) *The registration clerk should have been **authenticated** to use the system, and his or her authority to perform the registration task confirmed.*

   d) *Patients registering for procedures at the hospital are to be given a place with some privacy as they advise the clerk the reason for visit and their demographics. HIPAA permits "reasonableness" in compliance. Privacy compliance does not require a closed room; **reasonable** and appropriate measures must be provided to ensure confidential information is not easily overheard.*

4) Mrs. Goodman's primary care physician, Dr. Karing, is on the medical staff at the hospital. The Emergency Department gains access to Mrs. Goodman's records and prints out progress notes from her last office visit.

(continues)

(continued)

a) *The printer output must be protected from **unauthorized access**.*

b) *The progress notes are **protected health information**. All **individually identifiable health information** created, stored, or transmitted in both electronic and paper formats are specifically protected under HIPAA.*

c) *The Security Rule requires an **audit trail** showing who accessed the record and for what purpose and when. Although the rule does not specify the mechanics of the audit trail for paper, it is prudent to have a tracking mechanism for paper printouts and assign responsibility for monitoring their use and disposition.*

d) *The Security Rule requires **data backup and disaster recovery plan** (business continuity plan).*

5) A notation from the primary care physician, Dr. Karing, shows that Mrs. Goodman had seen a psychotherapist for depression. Dr. Eveready requests the psychotherapy notes to determine possible overdose of medications.

a) *HIPAA has special **authorization requirements** for **access to psychotherapy notes**. The general consent requirement for use and disclosure of **protected health information** for **treatment, payment, and health care operations** does not extend to psychotherapy notes. However, HIPAA allows for emergency access in circumstances where the patient is unresponsive.*

b) *A **business associate agreement** between Dr. Eveready and the psychotherapy facility is not required because Dr. Eveready is a provider who will use the information for treatment of Mrs. Goodman.*

c) *The psychotherapy facility must **authenticate** Dr. Eveready. The **minimum necessary** standard does not apply because Dr. Eveready is a health care provider requesting information to be used in treating Mrs. Goodman. All information excluded from psychotherapy notes is included in the usual progress notes retained by health care providers and do not need special authorization. See discussion in chapter 2, "Privacy Issues Explained," regarding disclosure of psychotherapy notes.*

6) The Emergency Department sees a prescription for medicine that could be used as a possible suicide drug. The Emergency Department requests STAT report, but the local hospital lab does not perform this test—it is sent to an outside lab.

a) *The Reference Lab does not have to provide a **Notice of Privacy Practices** to Mrs. Goodman even though they are a provider of services because it is an indirect provider.*

b) *A **business asssociate** contract is not required for reference lab because it is an indirect health care provider.*

7) The primary care physician's file that was accessed by the registration clerk indicates that Mayor Goodman has power of attorney for health care. The registration clerk phones the mayor's office to inform the mayor of his mother's status. The clerk talks with the mayor's assistant, who passes on the information that the mayor's mother has been taken to the hospital.

a) ***Disclosure of protected health information** is permitted to those who have been given authority to "stand in the patient's shoes" as **personal representatives** of the patient to exercise the patient's rights.*

b) ***Protected health information** must not be disclosed to anyone other than a patient or **personal representative**. The message should indicate that it is important for the mayor to call the hospital as soon as possible. Only general condition and location can be given to the assistant. The same would apply to a message left on an answering machine or voice mail.*

8) Ambulance personnel notify local authorities of their suspicion of elderly abuse based on information gained from the neighbor who called them, as well as viewing the unhealthy living conditions they found in Mrs. Goodman's home.

   a) *Information may be disclosed without Mrs. Goodman's authorization or Mayor Goodman's authorization if there is reason to believe patient has been a **victim of abuse, neglect, or domestic violence**.*

9) The patient's clinical information is entered into the hospital computer system by the Emergency Department staff and is displayed on a monitor in the Emergency Department's patient room.

   a) *Patient information is not to be available to anyone other than those involved in the treatment of the patient. The monitors cannot display **protected health information** so that other patients, family members, or employees and staff without the proper authority or the "**need to know**" can view it.*

10) The Emergency Department has trouble with their printer and calls the Information Services Department to fix it.

    a) *Since Information Services Department employees are employees of the hospital, they do not need a **business associate** agreement to repair equipment.*

    b) *If an outside firm is called in, then a **business associate** agreement is needed to ensure any repairperson will not disclose **protected health information** they saw while on site.*

11) Mrs. Elsa Goodman regains consciousness and her condition stabilizes. The Registration Department provides her with a **Notice of Privacy Practices**. Mrs. Goodman shakes her head that she does not want her hospitalization published—"**opting out**" of the directory listings. Staff asks if there is anyone she does wish to know of her condition. She mentions her son, the mayor. The hospital has a **policy** that allows patients to further restrict disclosure to the extent of anonymity, but she does not exercise that option.

    a) *The hospital must explain that her information will be put in the published **hospital directory** and allow her an opportunity to object.*

    b) *The hospital must provide her with a **Notice of Privacy Practices**. Consent to treat is not required by HIPAA but is often a **policy** of the provider.*

    c) *Once the option to **opt out** of the hospital directory is received, the hospital will not place Mrs. Goodman's name in a published listing of patients. This listing is often sent to a local newspaper and radio station for publication.*

    d) *Even though she **opted out** of the published listings, general information about condition and location may still be released if the asking party provides Mrs. Goodman's full name. This includes family.*

    e) *The facility may have stricter **policies** about anonymity, which would take **precedence**.*

12) Mrs. Goodman is sent to Radiology Department for X-rays of her arm and chest to check for probable fracture of her arm and other possible damage. She is also given a CAT scan of her head to determine possible cranial injury from the fall.

    a) *Radiology Department personnel must be **authenticated** by the system to access the patient database to add a report to Mrs. Goodman's medical record.*

(continues)

(continued)

b) *The Privacy Rule does not limit sharing of medical information for **reasons of treatment, payment, or health care operation**.*

c) *Any monitors, reports, or view boxes must be kept from public view in the Radiology Department because care must be taken not to disclose **protected health information** to anyone other than those directly treating the patient.*

d) *Radiology film must not be viewable or accessible in public areas. This is required by the **Privacy Rule**; the **Security Rule** also applies if information is in electronic form.*

13) An oblique closed fracture on the shaft of the ulna and an incomplete fracture of the tibia are found on X-rays. Mrs. Goodman is admitted to the hospital for surgery as well as observation. Arrangements are made for surgical staff, headed by Dr. Bones, the staff orthopedist, to reduce the fracture and apply casting. She will remain in the hospital for observation, possibly for two days, to ensure her condition is stable. No other fracture or other serious injury is noted. She does remain confused and disoriented.

a) *HIPAA allows **business as usual** as much as possible. There are no special **authorization** requirements for Dr. Bones to provide care.*

b) *Both doctors are known to each other through hospital contact and are credentialed with the hospital. There is no requirement for Dr. Eveready to have a **business associate** agreement with Dr. Bones.*

c) *There is no limit to disclose only "**minimum necessary**" information for purposes of **treatment**.*

d) *The physician and nursing staff can view all of the medical records since they need to understand her condition. Authorization is not necessary for reasons of **treatment, payment, or health care operations**.*

e) *The treating physician must be **authenticated** to use the computer system.*

f) *Any nursing staff that has information to chart about Mrs. Goodman's care must also be **authenticated** to use the computer system and log off appropriately.*

14) Before going into the OR, Dr. Bones consults with another orthopedist about the best means to reduce the fracture. The surgical staff gathers to review the procedure. The anesthesiologist, Dr. Bones, and the operating room nurses proceed with the surgery. They have views of the fractures provided through a PACS (Picture Archiving Communication System) maintained by the hospital.

a) *Any physician called in on a consulting basis must abide by the provisions of the **Privacy Rule** concerning all **protected health information** reviewed. Special authorization is not required since the disclosure is for normal **treatment, payment or health care operations**.*

b) *Any physician, anesthesiologist, nursing staff, LPN, or CNA who attends to Mrs. Goodman must abide by the provisions of the **Privacy Rule** and not disclose anything that could relate a diagnosis with the patient's identity. It is best if they do not chat idly about medical issues with anyone outside of the health care staff who are assigned to Mrs. Goodman's care. This would include staff in other departments within the facility.*

15) During surgery, the C-arm X-ray machine malfunctions. It requires a biomed technician to diagnose the reason for failure.

a) *If the hospital has a biomed technician on staff, that technician has been **trained** under HIPAA policies and understands the necessity to follow **policies** relating to **protected health information**.*

    b)   *If the hospital contracts with an outside firm for biomed services, there must be a **business associate** agreement in place prior to the technician coming in to diagnose the equipment.*

16)   The remainder of the surgery goes well without any complications, and Mrs. Goodman is moved to the recovery room. The Housekeeping Department is called to clean the OR suite. Housekeeping staff find one of the monitors still showing the results of the radiology X-rays through the PACS. The staff member calls to the nurse's station to have it shut down appropriately.

    a)   *Leaving protected health information open or available for others to view would be an **incidental disclosure** since the operating areas are not open to the public. It should be reported and logged into the patient record. The disclosure would be incidental since it is not considered an intentional distribution of **protected health information**. This is a violation of the **Privacy Rule** and the **Security Rule** since the information is in electronic format on the PACS.*

    b)   *If the information were in the form of X-ray films hung on the view box, the breach would be a violation of only the **Privacy Rule** since the **protected health information** is not electronic.*

17)   At break, a Surgical Department employee chats with other employees from various departments about their day. One of them mentions that the mayor's mother was brought in and that the staff wondered about her treatment and the mayor's upstanding position in the community. The discussion left those listening with questions about the mayor's family ethics.

    a)   *The Privacy Rule requires immediate action to remedy any disclosure except for reasons of **treatment, payment, or health care operations**. An employee should report concerns to his supervisor, HIPAA officer, or law enforcement officials at the Department of Health and Human Services, not the individual. The disclosure must be reported and corrected before it adversely affects the facility. Any whistle-blowing should be encouraged and protected within the organization, with steps taken to immediately remedy the incident. Unchecked, the ramifications can reach all the way to the CEO of the organization. All employees must comply with the HIPAA **Privacy Ruling** as specified by the health care provider's **policy** or face the consequences: either action under by the health care provider's **policy** or legal action against the health care provider by the Department of Health and Human Services. For the employee, it might include job termination.*

    b)   *A record of this **disclosure** must be added to the patient record when an employee reports it. This is true whether the disclosure is incidental or deliberate as described above.*

    c)   *The employee must be disciplined according to written **policies** as specified by the HIPAA Privacy Rule. Documentation is to be placed in the employee's file.*

18)   During a lull in the work schedule, an OB nurse who has access to the patient database uses the computer system to look through Mrs. Goodman's file.

    a)   *The computer system must have an **audit trail** that is kept for three years for all personnel who access information. The **audit trail** notes what is viewed, when, and whether anything has been changed in the record.*

    b)   *As with the Emergency Department employee, strong disciplinary action must be taken when those who do not "**need to know**" access **protected health information**.*

19)   Since word has gotten out that the patient is the mayor's mother, a local reporter comes to the information desk manned by auxiliary volunteers to ask about her condition. He asks for her by name.

(continues)

(continued)

a) *HIPAA allows* **release of directory information** *to the public. This includes patient's name, location in the facility, and description, in general terms, of the patient's condition. Local facility* **policy** *will instruct personnel about the extent of information available to reply to a request for patient information. It would be in the patient's best interest to insist the visitor give the full name of the patient, not only a surname or first name.*

b) *Some facilities issue passwords to individuals approved by the patient to receive more detailed information. This is a* **reasonable** *means to protect patients' privacy and protect the health care provider from liability.*

c) *Mrs. Goodman has* **opted-out** *of the facility directory so the journalist would have to ask for information using her full name.*

20) The next day, Mrs. Goodman's clergyman comes to the hospital to visit parishioners. He stops at the information desk to request a list of members of his denomination that are listed as inpatients.

a) *An individual's religious affiliation may be disclosed only to clergy if the patient has not objected to such disclosure.* **Opting out** *of the facility directory is not an objection to this disclosure. Any patient who has registered under a religious denomination is placed on the list by denomination. Visiting clergy who request information concerning patients listed under their denomination will be given a list with name, room location, and current status.*

b) *Since Mrs. Goodman has* **opted out**, *the facility may still have Mrs. Goodman's name on the denominational list as a patient who is available only to clergy. The denominational list is separate from and treated differently from the published directories. Disclosure to the clergy may be limited to denomination, name, and location in the facility.*

21) The hospital is a teaching hospital so medical interns participate in rounds with Dr. Eveready and report about Mrs. Goodman at "grand rounds."

a) *The* **definition of health care operations** *includes "conducting training programs in which students, trainees, or practitioners in areas of health care learn under supervision to practice or improve their skills as health care providers."*

b) *Medical students must be* **trained** *about HIPAA, and the education must be documented.*

c) *No special authorization is needed for this activity. It is permitted under "normal* **health care operations**."

22) Dr. Eveready consults with resident psychotherapist Dr. Wise, regarding patient's status and modification of meds to stabilize her condition if lab tests deem necessary.

a) *HIPAA does not limit disclosure of* **protected health information** *when it is for the treatment of a patient.*

23) The patient Accounts Department contacts Mrs. Goodman's health plan via online services to verify her eligibility using ASC X12N 270 and receives a response using ASC X12N 271 that her coverage is current and benefits provide for emergency care.

a) *The eligibility inquiry and response must follow the* **designated ASC X12N standard format**.

b) *The health plan, as a* **covered entity**, *may request* **minimum necessary** *information to process the request.*

c) *Specific authorization is not required since* **protected health information** *is disclosed for* **payment** *of services.*

d) *Any online transactions must be **encrypted** and a transmission log must be kept for three years.*

24) Dr. Bones dictates his operative report on Mrs. Goodman. After Dr. Bones signs using electronic signature software, the electronic report becomes part of her medical record.

 a) *If a transcription service is used, a **business associate** contract must be in place. They must have received **training** in HIPAA **Privacy** and **Security** issues and have that documented on file at the hospital.*

 b) *Information sent across the Internet must be **encrypted**.*

 c) *If transcription is done by hospital employees, those employees must also be **trained** in HIPAA **privacy** and **security** and have the training documented. This **training** must be kept on record for at least three years.*

 d) *Dr. Bones may use his electronic signature as long as the system **authenticates** him, integrity is maintained, and there is **nonrepudiation security**.*

 i) *Nonrepudiation: A 100 percent certainty that the physician did sign the document, making it legal. Conversely, it cannot be proven that the physician did not sign the report or document. The document is undeniably authentic.*

25) Local authorities, notified by Emergency Department personnel, request an interview with the patient to see if allegations about the possible abuse are founded.

 a) *HIPAA permits **disclosure of protected health information** to appropriate government authorities in cases of **victims of abuse, neglect, or domestic violence**. The agents may question the patient.*

26) By evening, the dietary staff brings up a meal for Mrs. Goodman.

 a) *Dietary staff may talk with the patient but cannot speak of her detailed condition to anyone. This is information they obtained as part of their work situation. These facts must be kept confidential under the **Privacy Rule**.*

27) The next day, housekeeping comes to clean the room and change bedclothes.

 a) *Like the dietary staff, housekeeping staff is not to reveal information about the condition of Mrs. Goodman. This is in keeping with the **Privacy Rule**. Keep in mind that local policy may be more restrictive.*

28) Dr. Eveready dictates Emergency Department notes and identifies diagnoses and procedures performed. A copy is placed in Dr. Eveready's records also for teaching purposes.

 a) *A teaching file must contain only **minimum necessary** information needed for teaching purposes.*

 b) *All possible **identifiers** must be eliminated from the record so it cannot be traced to a real patient.*

29) Software in the Emergency Department searches for candidates for a statewide research study about treatment of elderly by family and neighbors. A research coordinator arrives at the hospital, obtains an informed consent from Mrs. Goodman, and starts the research protocol.

 a) *Mrs. Goodman's authorization for participation in the **research study** is required under FDA regulations, not HIPAA.*

 b) *Clinical **research studies** can access patient information without authorization provided that an IRB or privacy board has approved the research protocol.*

(continues)

(continued)

    c) *Researchers may obtain properly **de-identified** clinical data without authorization.*

        i) *To be "**de-identified**," the data cannot contain any of 18 specific identifiers of an individual and his or her relatives, employers, or household members.*

        ii) *If any identifiers remain, the data may be released if a qualified statistician determines the risk of re-identification is very small.*

        iii) *Certain conditions in small communities may apply that require further **de-identification** to prevent deduced identification.*

30) Dr. Bones dictates his operative report. His office transcriptionist prepares it for the doctor's signature.

    a) *Like hospital transcriptionists, all doctors' staff must have **training** in HIPAA and have it documented in office files.*

31) Mrs. Goodman receives some physical therapy towards the end of her stay.

    a) *The Physical, Speech and Rehabilitation Therapy Departments are **covered entities** and do not need special **authorization** in order to treat patients.*

    b) *Their progress notes are entered into the medical record. The computer system must **authenticate** them to use the system through login and password access. They are given full access to the medical record since they are using it for treatment of a patient.*

32) Health Information Management Department (Medical Records) receives patient information and abstracts information for medical record and billing purposes. They prepare a tentative diagnosis-related group report on Mrs. Goodman. This advises the hospital of prospective reimbursement they will receive for the care of Mrs. Goodman.

    a) ***Disclosure of protected health information** is permitted for purposes of **treatment, payment, and health care operations**.*

33) After discharge and completion of all physician reports, the Patient Accounts Department submits their bill to a clearinghouse that checks the billing for errors and then forwards it to the patient's insurance company electronically, following HIPAA Transaction and Code Set ruling.

    a) *This transmission is a **designated ANSI X12 standard transaction**, N 837 Health Care Claim: Institutional, compliant with HIPAA transaction using **designated code sets** and **identifier standards**. The insurance company or health plan must accept the bill in this format and cannot deny payment because it was received electronically.*

    b) *The hospital may request status of the claim using a **standardized transmission request**, ANSI X12N 276. The health plan must reply using the **standardized transmission reply** format, ANSI X12N 277.*

    c) *Payment will most likely be processed electronically using **designated ANSI X12 standard format** N 835, Health Care Claim Payment Advice, into the hospital's account if there is nothing noted on the claim that would need review.*

    d) ***Health care clearinghouses** are **covered entities** and must treat **protected health information**, as does the hospital—with all privacy concerns. They are subject to all **privacy** and technical **security** standards of HIPAA.*

34) Dr. Bones's insurance billing specialist reviews the report, abstracts information for proper coding, and submits a CMS-1500 bill to the insurance company for Dr. Bones's services in

surgery. While the specialist is working on the file, the repairman for the office photocopier comes to fix the machine.

a) *The claim form is transmitted using **designated ANSI X12 standard format** 837. Software **encrypts** the claim as it is sent and the receiving party translates it back to legible format for processing.*

b) *The billing specialist is restricted to **minimum necessary** information to perform the job. If further information is needed for processing, the specialist should consult the clinical staff or a doctor who has no limitation on disclosure of information.*

c) *Any outside personnel who might see **protected health information** must have a **business associate's** written agreement. This protects patients from **incidental disclosure** of information while repairmen or additional personnel are on the premises for other purposes.*

35) Mr. Goodman is curious about what is written on his mother's medical record and requests a copy from the hospital for review. He has been named as "power of attorney for health care" by his mother.

a) *Patients or their representatives have the right to review and obtain a copy of a "**designated record set**" for as long as the **covered entity** maintains the information. The information disclosed must be defined by the extent of disclosure request, i.e., designated dates and type of information. A designated record set from a provider might include medical records or billing records. Information from a health plan might include enrollment records, payment records, claims adjudication records, or case management records.*

b) *There is no automatic right to access for psychotherapy notes; information in a criminal, civil, or administrative action; or **protected health information** exempted by the Clinical Laboratory Improvement Amendments.*

c) *A **covered entity** must act upon a request for information within 30 days, or 60 days if the information is off site.*

36) The mayor requests that the Health Information Management Department disclose to him who has received outside access to his mother's medical record.

a) *The **covered entity** must act on a request within 60 days with a possible 30-day extension.*

b) ***Written accounting of disclosures** of **protected health information must** include date of disclosure, person to whom the information was disclosed, brief description of information disclosed, and a copy of the authorization.*

c) ***Written accounting of disclosures** of **protected health information** are provided free once per year; charges may be included if more requests are received.*

d) *Documentation of **disclosures of protected health information must** be maintained for 6 years.*

37) Mr. Goodman asks to have the record changed because he believes it is not correct.

a) *Individuals, or their representatives, have the right to **request an amendment**, not change, as long as the **covered entity** maintains the information.*

b) *The **covered entity** may require a written request for rationale for the amendment and must act within 60 days of the request.*

c) *If the request is granted, the **covered entity** must*

    i) *notify the individual that the amendment was accepted.*

    ii) *inform relevant person(s) identified by the individual of the amendment.*

(continues)

(continued)

38) The hospital, after reviewing the request and discussing it with Dr. Eveready, denies the request to amend the medical record.

    a) *The **covered entity** may deny a request if **protected health information***

        i) *was not created by the **covered entity**.*

        ii) *is not part of the **designated record set** requested.*

        iii) *was not available for inspection.*

        iv) *was accurate and complete.*

    b) *The **covered entity** may prepare a rebuttal statement to the individual's statement of disagreement and must give a copy to the individual.*

39) After discharge from the hospital, Mrs. Goodman is to come to Dr. Eveready's office for a follow-up visit. Dr Eveready's receptionist calls the mayor's office to set up a follow-up appointment for Mrs. Goodman.

    a) *Since the mayor is Mrs. Goodman's **personal representative**, the doctor's receptionist can speak freely only with the mayor.*

    b) *If the mayor is not available to speak on the phone, the doctor's receptionist may leave a message with the mayor's assistant to have the mayor call the doctor's office, including the return phone number. The doctor's receptionist should communicate the **minimum necessary** information for the mayor to understand the request since his assistant is not the patient or authorized representative.*

40) The Hospital Foundation, following its usual custom, and considering the patient is mother of the town mayor, requests a contribution from the prominent family for expansion of the Emergency Department facility.

    a) *HIPAA rules permit this use of **protected health information** provided that notification of this type of use is included in its **Notice of Privacy Practices**.*

    b) *The family may **opt out** of future contact; how to do this must be included in the **Notice of Privacy Practices**.*

All the way through the process of treating, billing for services, and follow-up services, HIPAA has rulings concerning proper treatment of protected health information.

REVIEW QUESTIONS

1. What is the correct acronym for Public Law 104-191?

2. What government department has issued the details of HIPAA?

3. What are the four areas in which the federal law mandated changes in the protection of health information?

4. What issues forced Congress to pass HIPAA of 1996?

5. If HIPAA and state laws are different, which takes precedence? Are there any exceptions?

6. Define protected health information.

7. What part did the Department of Health and Human Services have in explaining the HIPAA law?

8. What are the two goals of the Title II: Administrative Simplification law?

9. List the three covered entities that must protect individually identifiable health information.

10. Discuss the difference between privacy and security of health information.

11. Why is it important to have an official HIPAA officer be part of compliance with the law?

12. Each health care facility must develop policies in relation to HIPAA. How would policies at each facility be different? How would they be the same?

REFERENCES

Appleby, J. (2002, March 23). File safe: Health records may no be confidential. *USA Today*, p. A1.

Are You a Covered Entity…and When Does Rule 1 Apply? (2001, August 24). *Road Maps to HIPAA Compliance* (Volume 2, Map 1. p. 7).

Covered Entity Charts, HIPAA General Information. (last modified December 14, 2005). Retrieved from http://www.cms.hhs.gov/HIPAAGenInfo/coveredentitycharts.pdf.

Health Insurance Portability and Accountability Act of 1996. (1996). H.R. 3103, 104th Cong.

HIPAA Electronic Transaction and Code Sets. (2003, March). Volume 1, Paper 1, Centers for Medicare and Medicaid Services, p.1.

HIPAA Readiness Checklist. (2003, March). Provider HIPAA checklist, moving toward compliance. *CMS HIPAA Electronic Transactions and Code Sets,* p.1.

Hobson, Hon, David L. (1997, October 23) *Clarification of the Health Information Portability and Accountability Act*, 105th Cong., E 2065. Retrieved March 20, 2003, from http://www.cms.hhs.gov/hipaa/hipaa2/general/bckground/hobson.asp.

McCarthy, E. (1999, April 5). Patients voice growing concerns about privacy. *Sacramento Business Journal*.

Medicare Program; Medicare Prescription Drug Benefit (Pub. L. 108-173). (January 28, 2005.) Federal Register, Vol. 70, No. 18, p. 4,201.

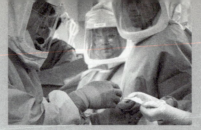

CHAPTER

2

PRIVACY ISSUES EXPLAINED

OBJECTIVES

Explain the definition of protected health information (PHI).

Recognize the difference between consent and authorization and their use in HIPAA.

Be familiar with required disclosures, those permitted without authorization, and those permitted with authorization

Identify when business associate contracts must be obtained.

Understand how HIPAA mandates training for the public and health care workforce.

Explain how the Department of Health and Human Services has ordered compliance with HIPAA law.

KEY TERMS

authorization

business associate (BA)

consent

de-identified health
  information

designated record set

disclosure (of protected
  health information)

emancipated minor

health care operations

health plan

incidental disclosure

individually identifiable
  health information
  (IIHI)

limited data set

marketing

minimum necessary

Office for Civil Rights
  (OCR)

opt out

psychotherapy notes

treatment

use (of protected health
  information)

workforce

INTRODUCTION

P rivacy of personal information is an important issue for everyone. Much personal information is being collected today. Stores track purchases by individual identification, banks and other financial organizations submit information to credit organizations to provide credit ratings, and closed-circuit cameras track many of our activities. With the move to protect our nation from terrorist activities, many enforcement agencies share information about individual activities. A federal rule about use of personal health information must have safeguards to protect private health information from being disclosed indiscriminately. The Department of Health and Human Services (DHHS) wrote the Privacy Rule to mandate nationwide standards to protect private health information.

THINK ABOUT IT

1. Why might someone not want their records copied and sent to their employer?
2. What could be included that would bias the employer against the worker?
3. What kind of information did patients receive from a health provider about their medical information after April 14, 2003?

TO WHOM DOES TITLE II APPLY?

The Health Insurance Portability and Accountability Act of 1996 (HIPAA), Public Law 104-191, was enacted on August 21, 1996. Title II of HIPAA has the title of Preventing Health Care Fraud and Abuse; Administrative Simplification; Medical Liability Reform. This is the portion that focuses on the health care industry. Title II, often referred to as Administrative Simplification, required the secretary of the DHHS to publicize standards for the privacy of all personal health information. The goal of the ruling was to protect information while still allowing the flow of health information needed to properly and effectively treat patients. The ruling was not intended to prevent health care givers from accessing information nor create situations that might bring harm to any patient through complicated steps of compliance. HIPAA clearly lists the circumstances when individual health information must be disclosed without an individual's authorization.

In April 2003, the first-ever federal privacy standards for medical data went into effect. Some states already regulated use and disclosure of medical records. There were many variations from state to state. Most doctors and clinical facilities realized that there needed to be limits on what information was released and to whom. Many people felt that their health information was open to anyone and everyone prior to April 2003. While this was not entirely true, as the vulnerability of electronic medical records became more widely known, people became very concerned. April 2003 was just the beginning of federal rulings to standardize how all patient information should be handled. With these rules in place, a person could travel anywhere in the United States and expect the same safeguards to be in place.

Privacy issues are administrative in nature. Each health care provider must have certain policies in place to comply with the rulings. This mandate includes all health care providers whether or not they transmit health claims electronically. Many of these policies and practices are not different from established clinical practices. Privacy compliance requires training staff to understand the rulings. Employees must follow certain policies for all the health care information they encounter in their work. Each health care facility must have written policies available to all employees for reference. If the **Office for Civil Rights (OCR)** conducts an investigation, the inspectors will expect to see written or electronic health care facility policies and procedures. If policies are on paper *and* in electronic form, they will likely assume that the electronic system is not to be trusted. In such a case, they will expect to see the printed policy handbook. Though the guidelines seem strict, HIPAA allows for a great deal of flexibility. The Privacy Rule allows each organization to do "what is reasonable" within the guidelines. The rule does not specify how to comply. For example, to prevent conversations from being overheard does not mean every time a physician speaks with a patient they must be in a room with the door closed. Reasonable and professional courtesy suggests that the physician ask visitors to leave the room or ask the patient if his or her care may be discussed with others present. As long as reasonable care is taken to comply with the intent of the ruling, and the reasonable effort is documented, that will be sufficient.

Appendix B has a listing of the Centers for Medicare and Medicaid (CMS) Regional Offices as well as other sources for HIPAA information. A number of health organizations conduct seminars to help interpret rulings and any revisions of the rulings. Local seminars will help staff connect with others in their field. Networking and sharing of ideas with other local health care providers is another valuable source of ideas.

What Is Protected Health Information?

An efficient way to determine if health information is to be protected is to consider if there can be an *association between the health condition and the individual.* If a name or other identifier can be connected with a health condition, diagnosis, or financial status, then that information comes under the HIPAA Privacy Rule and must be protected. The long definition for protected health information (PHI) is all *individually-identifiable health information* (IIHI) held or transmitted by or to a covered entity in any form or media, whether electronic, paper, or oral. A good understanding of what PHI encompasses will greatly help to understand when disclosure needs to be authorized. PHI may be any combination of a name, an address, social security number or other identification number, an insurance policy number, diagnosis, a procedure, or any **psychotherapy notes**. A complete definition of these notes will follow later in this chapter. Any single element listed by itself is *not* PHI. A diagnosis alone, an insurance account number alone, or a name alone does not fulfill this definition. General information that cannot be linked to a particular person does not come under this definition either. A caregiver is permitted to release the location of a patient and her general condition. For example, "She is in the ICU in critical condition," is permitted. Not permitted is the information that she was taken to the ICU because her diabetes became acute.

TRUE STORY

The medical records of an Illinois woman were posted on the Internet without her knowledge or consent a few days after she was treated at St. Elizabeth's Medical Center, following complications from an abortion at the Hope Clinic for Women. The woman has sued the hospital, alleging St. Elizabeth's released her medical records without her authorization to anti-abortion activists, who then posted the records online along with a photograph they had taken of her being transferred from the clinic to the hospital. The woman is also suing the anti-abortion activists for invading her privacy. (Hillig and Mannies, 2001).

Clearly, in the above story, this woman's privacy was violated in a number of ways. Perhaps this became a news report for a local journalist. However, the diagnosis or reasons for the transfer and hospital stay are not to be released without proper patient authorization. Directory information may be released but only that which verifies location within the facility and general condition of any patient.

HIPAA sets a minimum standard for privacy. Personal identifiers of any kind are the targets of identity thieves today. Every health care provider needs to carefully protect all personal information to prevent any opportunity for loss, theft, or unauthorized alteration. Each organization should have policies in place that address the protection of all personal information, whether HIPAA protected health information or not. This means both medical and financial records.

There are subtle ways that PHI can be disclosed. A location in a nursing home may indicate that a group of rooms are for Alzheimer's patients only, or hospital rooms may be only allotted to patients who are HIV positive. If patient names are displayed on these rooms, that constitutes a disclosure of PHI. The definition of **disclosure of protected health information (PHI)** is the release, transfer, divulging of, or providing access to PHI to an outside entity. This is different from use of PHI. The **use of PHI** is the sharing, employment, application, utilization, examination, or analysis of individually identifiable health information (IIHI) within an entity that maintains such information. The main difference between these definitions is where the information will end up—inside or outside the covered entity.

PHI is more than electronically transmitted health information. Under the Privacy Rule, the entire health record of any patient is covered. Included as PHI are radiology film with reports of ultrasounds, magnetic resonance imaging (MRI), computerized axial tomography (CAT) scans, tracings or tape printouts from stress tests, any laboratory reports, videotapes of the patient, audio reports or notes, rehabilitation department notes, dictation tapes, nurse's notes, nursing home files, and home health and public health nurse records. PHI may be held by a variety of health care providers. The list may include dentists, chiropractors, optometrists, opticians, morticians, school nurses, nursing homes, home health offices, clinics, and hospitals.

Individually identifiable health information (IIHI) is any demographic information about an individual that can possibly identify that individual. This could be full or partial name, address, social security number, birth date, or phone number. It can also include a description of someone's past, present, or future physical or mental health or condition; or past, present, or future payments for providing health care to an individual. In some cases, a zip code is an identifier. If all identification is eliminated from the record, and tracing of the individual is not possible, then the HIPAA ruling calls this **de-identified health information**. The best way to de-identify information is to remove all specified identifiers of the individual as well as any information concerning an individual's relatives, household members, and employers. Once this is done, then chances of knowing who the specific individual is will be quite incidental.

Authorization versus Consent

We have talked about authorization. What does authorization mean? How does it differ from the definition of consent? The patient who comes into the doctor's office and asks for treatment is giving implied consent for treatment. Some providers use the term "consent" to mean permission to treat, and have written policies requiring consent. **Consent** as defined by the original wording of HIPAA law is more than agreement to receive treatment. It gives permission to reveal PHI to other health care providers or covered entities in the process of comprehensive **treatment**, payment of services, and normal **health care operations**. Consent is not required by HIPAA for *treatment, payment, and normal business operations*. This is referred to as TPO—treatment, payment, and operations. HIPAA does not regulate the use of consent for treatment because the regulation of consent was removed from the final rule.

Authorization gives permission to disclose PHI for *reasons other than treatment, payment, or health care operations*. Authorization must include several very specific elements. Authorization for disclosure of PHI must be in writing. It must be in plain language. Authorization gives the covered entity permission to reveal specified health care information or a **designated record set**. The designated record set carefully describes the extent of information to be released. An example is a doctor's progress notes for a specified date range, or a radiology report and film taken on a certain date, or perhaps the complete medical record for the past three years. Authorization names the covered entity authorized to disclose information and the name of the entity or person to receive the information. The purpose of the disclosure is given and expiration of the permission is stated. Proper authorization includes a statement of the individual's right to revoke the authorization or reference to the covered entity's Notice of Privacy Practices, which includes that information. Authorizations must include a statement that information may be subject to redisclosure by the recipient and is then no longer protected by federal law. Finally, it must be signed by the individual or their legal representative and dated. A health care provider worker should verify the identity of the individual requesting release of information, preferably with photo identification. This format has been used in most Health Information Management Departments prior to HIPAA.

TRUE STORY

Consider how not authorizing release of information changed this woman's employment status. Why might employers want to know medical history of employees? Are these valid reasons?

A South Carolina resident was suspended from work for refusing to release her medical records to her employer. (Crowley, 2000).

TABLE 2-1   Contrast difference between consent and authorization

	Consent	Authorization
Purpose	For T P O (treatment, payment, and health care operations)	For other than T P O
Required by HIPAA	No	Yes
Written	Not necessary per HIPAA; can be specified by health care provider policy	Yes, signed and dated
Released to	Entity who has a relationship with the individual for treatment, payment or normal business operations	Party specified in authorization other than a provider, health plan or clearinghouse

Health plans have information about the enrollment, payment, claims adjudication, and case or medical management record systems for the individuals covered by their plan. This information, which is not part of the health care provider's medical records, may only be disclosed with proper authorization. Table 2-1 shows the differences between consent and authorization.

THINK ABOUT IT

1. When more than one doctor is treating a patient, is a signed authorization needed in order to send the medical record to the other provider? If not, then what is required?
2. A health care provider discloses protected health information to a health plan for the plan's Health Plan Employer Data and Information Set (HEDIS) purposes. This health plan has a relationship with the individual who is the subject of the information. Is authorization needed? Should there be any limit to the disclosure?

Concerns about Protected Health Information and Possible Disclosures

The purpose of the Privacy Rule is to define and limit the circumstances in which an individual's PHI may be used or disclosed by covered entities. (OCR Privacy Rule Summary, 2003). It is noteworthy to understand that the OCR will investigate any complaint received. However, unless the infraction is considered serious, the intent of the investigation will be to correct and adjust policies and procedures so that compliance with the ruling is achieved.

Required Disclosures

The Privacy Rule requires covered entities to disclose PHI under *two conditions*. The first is when an individual requests access to his or her

TABLE 2-2 When PHI may be disclosed as defined in HIPAA

	Disclosure to:	Purpose of Disclosure
#1	Individual who requests access	Designated record set
#2	DHHS	Complete record for compliance purposes
#3	Legal authorities as defined by state law	Suspected neglect, abuse, domestic violence

medical records. The second required disclosure is when the DHHS comes to review records in regard to a compliance investigation. All other situations have limitations of various types. In most states, disclosure in the case of suspected neglect, abuse, or domestic violence is mandatory. This disclosure is listed as disclosure for public interest and to benefit the public and does not need authorization. Table 2-2 shows when PHI may be disclosed as defined by HIPAA.

Permitted Use and Disclosure without Authorization

The Privacy Ruling specifies six circumstances for permitted use and disclosure of health information *without authorization.* They are the following:

1. To the individual whose health information it is

2. For treatment, payment, and health care operations (TPO)

3. With opportunity to agree or object, for inclusion in directory, and disclosure to specified family members

4. Incidental to a permitted use and disclosure

5. For public interest and to benefit the public

6. For research and public health purposes without the identifiable information

For Individual Access

Individuals wishing to see their medical records are permitted to have access to the medical information about them. This includes parents, guardians, or other persons acting in loco parentis with legal authority to make health care decisions on behalf of minor children. Certain individuals may designate a "personal representative." This person legally "stands in the shoes" of the individual and has the power to authorize disclosures of health information as well. (Personal Representatives, 2002). When someone else is authorized to act for the patient, there are rules determining who that person can be and to what extent he or she can function. Table 2-3 shows how to recognize the personal representative in each category.

TABLE 2-3   Personal representative defined for various situations

If the Individual is: An Adult or An *Emancipated Minor*	*The Personal Representative is:* A person with legal authority to make health care decisions on behalf of the individual.	*Example:* Health care power of attorney, court appointed legal guardian, general power of attorney
If the Individual is: An Un-emancipated minor	*The Personal Representative is:* A parent, guardian or other person acting *in loco parentis* with legal authority to make health care decisions on behalf of the minor child.	*Example:* Parent of a minor child, guardian of a minor child or personal representative of a minor child. Certain exceptions apply—see Limiting Uses/Disclosures.
If the Individual is: Deceased	*The Personal Representative is:* A person with legal authority to act on behalf of the decedent or the estate (not restricted to health care decisions.)	*Example:* Executor of the estate, next of kin or other family member, durable power of attorney

*Note: An **emancipated minor** is someone under the age of eighteen (18) who lives independently and is totally self-supporting.*

For Treatment, Payment, and Health Care Operations

The second permitted use and disclosure of PHI that does not require authorization is for *treatment, payment, and health care operations.* This broad permission includes any and all services provided by one or more health care providers. Most of the PHI flows just as it did prior to HIPAA mandates. Doctors may share information concerning treatment and care of a patient. No limitation is placed on the *use* of PHI within a health care facility for the purposes of treating an individual. HIPAA also allows without authorization the *disclosure* of information between health care providers who are directly involved in treating or consultation with a particular patient. In certain circumstances, this disclosure may be to a health care provider who is not a covered entity. A primary care provider, who is a covered entity under the Privacy Rule, may send a copy of an individual's medical record to a specialist who needs the information to treat the same individual, whether or not that specialist is also a covered entity. No authorization or consent would be required. General psycho-therapy notes for treatment and payment as well as psychotherapy health care operations require an authorization *prior* to disclosure. Psychotherapy notes must be treated specially. We will address this later in this chapter.

Disclosures of PHI to a health plan in order to receive reimbursement for a service is permitted under HIPAA without further authorization. A health plan may request information to fulfill the responsibilities of the insurance policy. Any requests of a health plan to obtain premiums, pay claims, and fulfill the responsibilities of the insurance policy are permit-ted. The sharing of information to receive payment for services should be limited to the **"minimum necessary"** concept. The complete medical record or even the complete operative report is not necessary to verify that specific services were performed. Specific authorization is not required by HIPAA to disclose that data for payment. This is also true for payers who may not be covered entities—such as automobile or liability insurers. The deciding factor has to do with whether or not both entities have a relationship with the individual.

HIPAA states that there is no need for authorization for *normal health care operations*. This allows a very broad interpretation of what are normal operations. Permitted health care operations may include:

- Quality assessment and improvement activities
- Population-based activities relating to improving health care costs
- Case management
- Fraud and abuse detection and compliance programs
- Training programs
- Business planning and management
- Accreditation, certification, licensing, or credentialing activities
- Audits and legal services
- Certain fundraising activities of the business

Given the broad application of the term "authorization," the Office for Civil Rights has refined the ruling to emphasize the covered entity's responsibility to disclose only the *minimum necessary* to fulfill the request. (Standards for Privacy, 2002).

THINK ABOUT IT

A physician sends an individual's health plan coverage information to a laboratory that needs the information to bill for services it provided to the physician with respect to the individual. Is authorization needed?

When Permission to Disclose is Received

The third permitted use and disclosure of PHI is when *an individual is asked outright for authorization* to disclose certain information. When patients are admitted to a hospital facility, it is now a practice to ask if the patient would allow contact information to be published in the facility directory. Under the Privacy Rule, a provider may disclose the individual's general condition and his or her location within the facility to anyone who requests information *by name*. Often informal permission is granted to allow family and friends to be told the condition and location of a patient when asked for information by name. It must be documented that this authorization was verbal. That does not allow for someone to ask for "Somebody, I think his last name is Maxwell." They must give a complete name in order for information to be disclosed. When answering a phone call, one cannot prove that a caller is who they say they are. Health care facility personnel are required to make every reasonable effort to verify the identity of the inquirer. Be sure to document the request and the verification effort. When a visitor comes in person, it is reasonable to ask for some identification, preferably a photo ID. This permission is some-what informal and is considered *what is reasonable* but still protects the patient's privacy. This informal permission also allows a pharmacist to dispense prescriptions to a person acting on behalf of the patient.

THINK ABOUT IT

A "relative" calls the office and asks for a copy of "Mom's" lab report to be faxed to her house in order to take it to another doctor for a second opinion. Is this permitted under the Privacy Rule?

When Incidental

Incidental disclosures are the fourth permitted use of an individual's PHI. There will be times when there may be a disclosure of individually identifiable health information (IIHI). When this occurs as a result of or as "incident to" otherwise permitted use or disclosure, it is considered incidental. Reasonable safeguards must be in place to prevent this type of disclosure from happening regularly, but if it happens as incidental, there will be no penalty. For example, if a doctor is talking to a patient privately, but the conversation is overheard in spite of precautions like closing the door, the disclosure is considered *incidental*.

For Public Interest or to Benefit the Public

There are many disclosure possibilities allowed under the *public interest or to benefit the public* disclosure permit. Briefly, there are twelve national priority purposes for disclosure without an individual's authorization.

1. As *required by law*, under specific state law, or when ordered by a court.

2. To *control and/or prevent disease, injury, or disability by public health authorities*. This includes communicable diseases and work-related illnesses or accidents. This allows public health authorities to monitor trends.

3. In reporting *victims of abuse, neglect, or domestic violence.* The Privacy Rule states that when a physician or other health care provider reasonably believes that the individual, *whether an unemancipated minor or not,* has been subject to domestic violence, abuse, or neglect by the parent or personal representative, the health care provider may exercise professional judgment and *not* disclose certain health information to the parent or personal representative. This follows standards that many states already have in place. The ruling brings a national standard to releasing PHI in domestic violence, abuse, or neglect cases. A health care provider is legally responsible to report such cases to the appropriate authority. This might be the social services department of a local government. The police department is legally responsible when there is a possibility of criminal action. Whether or not the parent or family member is permitted to receive reports of health information is then up to the agency handling the case.

4. For *health oversight activities,* such as audits and investigations for oversight of the health care system and government benefit programs.

5. When requested by a *judicial or administrative tribunal,* or a subpoena from the courts.

6. For *law enforcement* purposes to identify a suspect or missing person; for information about a victim or suspect; to alert law enforcement of a person's death if the death is suspected to be as a result of a criminal act; when the PHI is evidence of a crime or assists in law enforcement investigations.

7. Information such as identification of deceased or to determine the *cause of death* may be disclosed to funeral directors or coroners.

8. PHI may be used to facilitate *donation and transplantation of organs, eyes, or tissue from deceased donors.*

9. When an institutional review board (IRB) or similar organization approves *research,* PHI may be released under strict guidelines. The guidelines limit the usage to strictly research purposes. It is expected that all information provided to the research organization be de-identified.

10. If there is believed to be a *serious threat to the health or safety of a person or the public,* covered entities may disclose PHI to civil or law enforcement authorities.

11. Certain *essential governmental functions* have authority to receive PHI. These instances may be assuring proper execution of a military mission, providing protective services to the president, or protecting the health and safety of inmates or employees of a correctional institution.

12. *Workers compensation laws* and other similar programs have permission to receive an individual's PHI in regard to work-related injuries or illnesses.

THINK ABOUT IT

The district attorney calls the office with a request that all documentation relating to a patient be released to her office. Is authorization needed? In what form should it be?

For Research

The last permitted disclosure of PHI is when a **limited data set** has been *de-identified for research purposes.* A limited data set is PHI from which certain specified direct identifiers of individuals and their relatives, household members, and employers have been removed. In other words, de-identified health information may be used for research or public health purposes with the understanding that specific safeguards are in place so information cannot be tied to an individual. This includes removing zip codes of areas with a population under 10,000 people.

Permitted Use and Disclosure with Authorization

The federal ruling has specified two situations when it is permitted to disclose PHI if given proper authorization. One instance is for the notes taken by a psychotherapist. The medical information shared within the confines of the psychotherapist's office needs special consideration, and the parties involved must have a clear understanding of what the government permits and what must be protected. The other permitted use is for purposes of marketing. Many businesses wish to enhance their profits by contacting potential customers. The proper use of PHI for marketing purposes is outlined carefully in the Privacy Rule.

Disclosure of Psychotherapy Notes

When it comes to psychotherapy notes, many states have regulations that already limit their release. Again, the HIPAA Privacy Rule supplements those regulations and limits the release of any notes or health information under this category. Special authorization is needed unless the information is to be used for treatment, payment, or health care operations.

The DHHS has issued clarification about the definition of psychotherapy notes. These are more often referred to as *process notes.* They capture the therapist's impressions about the patient. They often contain details considered to be inappropriate for the medical record. These process notes are kept separate within the medical office to limit access, even in an electronic records system. (Psychotherapy Notes, 2000). However, summary information, such as the current state of the patient, medication prescription and monitoring, side effects, counseling sessions start and stop times, the modalities and frequencies of treatment furnished, results of clinical tests, and any summary of the diagnosis, functional status, treatment plan, symptoms, prognosis and progress to date, and other information necessary for treatment or payment, is always placed in the patient's medical record. (OCR Privacy Rule Summary, 2003). Summary information is routinely sent to insurers for payment and is treated as other PHI.

Psychotherapy notes may be used within the covered entity for treatment of their patient. A covered entity may also defend itself legally and use the PHI in its defense. Psychotherapy notes can be used by the DHHS to investigate compliance with the Privacy Rule. Disclosure is permitted under HIPAA when there appears to be a serious or imminent threat to public health or safety. In this case, health information can be made known to appropriate authorities to protect the individual or the general population.

Disclosure for Marketing Purposes

The Privacy Rule allows for PHI to be used in certain ways for **marketing** purposes. When a marketing arrangement is made between two parties, there is an exchange of direct or indirect payment. Health care facility or hospital workers may ask a patient in person if they may speak about some promotion, gifts, or product they might recommend. If verbal permission is granted, it is considered authorization and should be documented. Otherwise, PHI cannot be released for marketing purposes, with these four exceptions.

1. The patient may receive information about health-related products or services that are included in an insurance coverage.

2. Communication about enhancements to a health insurance plan or related services to add to the patient's coverage may be directed to a member of the health plan.

3. A health care provider may communicate various options to an individual for consideration for treatment.

4. Communication may occur for the case management and coordination of a patient. In addition, information may be given to an individual concerning alternative treatments, therapies, or care settings (such as temporary rehabilitation facilities).

THINK ABOUT IT

Consider in the following situations whether HIPAA defines the scenario as marketing.

A. An endocrinologist shares a patient's medical records with several behavior management programs to determine which program best suits the ongoing needs of the individual patient. Is this considered marketing?

B. A health plan sells a list of its members to a manufacturing company that sells blood glucose monitors. This manufacturer intends to send the plan's members brochures on the benefits of purchasing and using the monitors. Is this considered marketing?

C. Consider a mailing from a health insurer promoting a home and casualty insurance product offered by the same company. Is this considered marketing?

Disclosure for Directory Purposes

One of the most misunderstood items in the Privacy Rule is the requirement to allow patients to **"opt out"** of the published directory listings. Upon registration, the patient must be asked about including his or her name in the published patient lists. If a patient "opts out," it should not be interpreted as a wish to remain anonymous, have no contact with visitors, or be kept in secrecy. HIPAA allows covered entity policy to be more restrictive than the law actually states. All HIPAA is protecting is the option to disallow participation in published lists. When a patient "opts out," it would be a good idea to clarify if he or she wants secrecy or if there are individuals the patient wants informed of his or her condition. Other facility rules may allow for complete anonymity for particular patients.

Clergy, and clergy only, may view the religious affiliation list of patients. It is permitted for clergy members to be told of the patients who have listed their religious affiliation as the same as the clergy member's. For example, a Methodist clergyman is permitted to view the list of patients whose religious affiliation is also listed as Methodist unless the patients have chosen to not be in the denominational lists. "Opting out" of the facility's published directory does not mean the patient has automatically "opted out" of the denominational list also.

Limiting Uses and Disclosures

Certain exceptions to the Privacy Rule apply to parents and unemancipated minors. The Privacy Rule prohibits a health care provider from disclosing a minor child's PHI when and to the extent that it is expressly prohibited under state or other laws. The Privacy Rule lists three circumstances when

PHI is to be withheld from the parent of an unemancipated minor. The three exceptions are as follows:

1. When a state or other law does not require parental consent and the minor consents to the heath care service. In this instance, the Privacy Rule states that parents do not have the right to certain health information.

2. When a court determines that someone other than the parent is allowed to make decisions concerning the medical treatment of a minor.

3. When a parent agrees to a confidential relationship between the minor and the physician. In this situation, if the physician asks the parent(s) if she can speak confidentially with an adolescent child about a medical condition and the parent(s) agree, then that information is restricted from the parents. (OCR Privacy Rule Summary, 2003).

Minimum Necessary Uses

In all of these situations, the Privacy Rule holds to the premise that only the "minimum necessary" PHI is disclosed. A complete record of a patient would probably be too much information and not be authorized for most purposes. This includes disclosure to the DHHS for investigation of a complaint, or as required by HIPAA law or other state or local laws. For example, a doctor providing care to a patient is able to access the patient's complete medical record history on demand.

In order to comply with the HIPAA ruling, any covered entity must develop a list of persons within their **workforce** who will have complete access to PHI, who else has limited access, and *the extent of that access*. It is expected that each health care facility knows the *minimum necessary* information for each position within the workforce. The HIPAA privacy officer would be the person that oversees this aspect of compliance. She is to provide safeguards that limit the access as outlined. A receptionist would need certain information in order to schedule appointments and would understand the time needed for each patient's appointment. The receptionist does not need to know details and have access to the progress notes made for each patient. That information, however, is important for the nursing staff, doctor, and the coding person in the Medical Records Department. The medical office assistant who does the billing will not need to see the complete medical record. When a claim is in question due to medical necessity, the claim should be referred to those individuals who have access to the complete information for adjustments.

THINK ABOUT IT

As part of a workers compensation claim case in California, John Doe authorized that his medical records be released. Doe's HIV status was revealed in the process, even though it was not relevant to the case. Despite the existence of a strong HIV confidentiality law in California, the court ruled that there was no obligation to segregate the information. (California Appellate Court, 2000).

a.   How does HIPAA address this?
b.   What could be part of the authorization that might prevent this full disclosure?

BUSINESS ASSOCIATES UNDER THE PRIVACY RULE

Scenario: Consider a repairperson coming to your office to work on the facsimile machine. Would she have access to any protected health information in order to repair the machine? Would any information in the memory of the machine be information that should be restricted? Some arrangement must be in place to insure that any PHI that the repairperson might encounter while on your premises is properly handled by the repairperson. That agreement is called a business associate agreement.

The Privacy Rule defines a **business associate (BA)** as a person or organization that performs or assists a function or activity on behalf of a covered entity, but is not part of the covered entity's workforce. A BA can also be a covered entity in its own right. Functions may involve the use or disclosure of PHI, including claims processing, data analysis, administration, utilization review, quality assurance, billing, benefit management, practice management, and repricing, or providing legal, actuarial, accounting, consulting, accreditation, or financial service to or for a covered entity.

These jobs might include processing insurance claims or servicing copiers. It would also include contractors doing the coding for claims or fixing a biometric device that contains PHI. Transcriptionists working as contractors are BAs, as are legal advisors for a doctor, clinic, or hospital. BAs are those who may not have direct contact with the patient or PHI but who access PHI incidentally in order to do their job. These people may not be directly involved with patient care yet are necessary to run the business part of the organization. Another category of BA is the vendors who provide equipment and supplies to the covered entity. A copy machine repairperson or delivery person should not be directly exposed to PHI, but she may have incidental access or be unattended. A BA agreement with such vendors will protect the health care provider. Refer to the Appendix B for a sample of Business Associate Contract Provisions as printed by the Office for Civil Rights. This is also available from the Web site for the OCR at http://www.hhs.gov/ocr.

TRAINING OF THE PUBLIC AND WORKFORCE

As of April 2003, all clinical offices, hospitals, clinics, eye doctors, chiropractors, specialists, and anyone who has records of any health information are required by the Privacy Rule to provide each patient with a Notice Of Privacy Practices (NOPP). Every health care provider who makes a direct face-to-face contact with a patient is required to obtain from the patient a written acknowledgment of the receipt of these privacy notices. The NOPP cannot be summarized and offered to the patient. The disclosure of the NOPP *must* be complete. A signed receipt for the NOPP must be in a patient's record. This signature is optional, but there must be a "good faith effort" to get a signature. If signature is refused, this only indicates that there has been an objection to the notice. This refusal should be documented and placed in the patient's file. This does not give the provider cause to refuse treatment. Consent to treat is a separate concept and not required by HIPAA. The fact that the patient has made an appointment and showed up for the appointment is implied consent to treat.

There are six elements each health care facility must disclose to their patients in the Notice Of Privacy Practices.

1. The ways they use and disclose PHI

2. Their duties to protect patient's privacy

3. A notice of their practices to ensure a patient's privacy

4. The terms of the current notice

5. Individual rights concerning PHI

6. A means of contacting the health care facility for further information or to place a complaint (OCR Privacy Rule Summary, 2003)

THINK ABOUT IT

A surgeon's office often contacts the hospital and other health care providers to collect pre-op information over the phone. This aids the surgeon in determining if there are medical concerns to be addressed prior to surgery. The patient has not received the Notice Of Privacy Practices as yet. Does the Privacy Rule prohibit this disclosure since the patient has not signed a NOPP receipt from this surgeon?

The **HIPAA officer** has the responsibility to see that each new employee is trained in HIPAA policy and procedures. Records of this training are to be kept for six years—the statute of limitations for civil penalties. HIPAA also expects to find records showing a yearly review of HIPAA policies for every employee. The office would need to possibly retrain employees when they move to a different department because the need for access to PHI could change. The employees must be trained for that new responsibility. (Requirements for Policies and Procedures, and Documentation Requirements, 2000). Periodic retraining is mentioned in the HIPAA law. Scheduling yearly review is appropriate and ensures that all employees have been reminded of requirements of the law.

Amending Protected Health Information

The Privacy Rule gives patients a right to access only their personal medical records. They can obtain a copy of their records. The original belongs to the agent or health care facility that created them. This ruling also gives anyone the right to *amend* his or her medical record by appending it. This is an addition to, not a change of, their record. If a patient disagrees with something in her record, she may add to the record written comments or other documentation of her choosing. A patient may add information that she feels is missing. However, a covered entity has the option to deny this request to amend the record. In this case, the individual is permitted to submit a statement of disagreement and have that statement of disagreement included in the medical record. This option of viewing and possibly amending one's medical record is not a new procedure. The federal government has now made a uniform ruling about how this can be done in any state.

With more and more identity theft, there comes the problem of correcting one's medical record that has been used by another. The damage left behind on the medical record as a result of stolen health care can have very devastating consequences to the individual for future treatment and proper coverage of benefits. Similar damage to the permanent record can occur through errors within the health care facility itself.

The author had a near-miss situation develop during a stay in a hospital. A caregiver came to administer a diabetes blood test. The author is not diabetic and was not alert enough to know what was happening. No names were called out, nor were ID bands scanned. If an alert bystander, in this case a patient-advocate wife, had not challenged the caregiver effectively, the results of the test would have been assigned to the wrong person, creating a bad outcome potential for both parties. In this case, an amendment would only add to the medical record but not expunge the error from the record. Certain measures need to be taken in the record to mark any false health information as incorrect when the health care provider agrees to the amendment. Correcting this bad information in a permanent medical record is beyond the scope of HIPAA, but HIPAA does help by giving the individual access to the record for review and the option of amending it.

It should be noted that identity theft and health care services theft are not directly addressed by HIPAA. They are covered by other civil codes and penalties that predate HIPAA. HIPAA expects a health care provider, compliant with HIPAA, to be proactive against such thievery, if for no other reason than awareness. It is prudent for an organization to consider risks of identity and health care services theft as separate items and take appropriate action.

The Privacy Rule also allows a patient the option of restricting who receives access to their PHI. Individuals have the right to see a listing of disclosures, authorized or not. This listing does not include disclosures for treatment, payment, and health care operations (TPO), which are normal and routine access necessary to conduct business.

The DHHS understands that the Privacy Rule must be flexible to meet all sizes of covered entities. The ruling is written so that each provider can implement the Privacy Rule to meet the needs of its own particular situation. The DHHS *does expect* each provider to have 1) written policy and procedures, 2) a privacy official within the organization, and 3) a workforce that is trained to comply with the ruling. Everyone employed is expected to know where to find the policies of that facility. They may be written and kept current in a policy book located in the department. The policies may be available electronically through intranet or Internet access rather than on paper. The workers are also expected to understand how the policies affect their particular areas of work. An important expectation of the DHHS is that a provider may not retaliate against a person for exercising her rights to question policy or report an unauthorized disclosure. Each organization must have appropriate safeguards in place to prevent disclosure of PHI and a means to relieve or resolve any harmful effect that might be caused if an inappropriate disclosure of PHI has occurred. Each covered entity must maintain its privacy policies and procedures for at least six years after their creation.

ENFORCEMENT GUIDELINES

The main intent of enforcement is *not* to criminally punish or impose fines. Strong enforcement from the OCR will be evident when there is blatant and obvious disregard for the ruling and resistance to correcting the problem. Noncompliance with the Privacy Rule does bring civil penalties and possibly criminal penalties if the violation is severe. The DHHS seeks to foster cooperation with the ruling rather than impose penalties. According to the *Fort Worth Star-Telegram*, 19,240 grievances have been lodged nationwide as of June 5, 2006. More than 73 percent (more than 14,000) of the grievances have been closed either by ruling that there was no violation or by allowing accused entities to promise better compliance. Of the 5,000 remaining cases as of June 2006, 309 have been referred to the Department of Justice as possible criminal violations.

(Stein, 2006). "These offices have worked for compliance. Winston Wilkinson, head of the Office for Civil Rights said, 'Our first approach to dealing with any complaint is to work for voluntary compliance. So far, it's worked out pretty well.'" (Stein, 2006). This is consistent with earlier comments about enforcement plans attributed to DHHS and accounts for the quick dispatch of so many grievances as noted above. It appears that most entities have taken the actions required for compliance. A survey by American Health Information Management Association (AHIMA) showed in 2004 that the most common problems appear to be lack of standardized processes for release of PHI and public access to records. Other common problems are the following:

1. Accounting for release of PHI

2. Obtaining PHI from other providers

3. Accessing and releasing of information to relatives or spouse

4. Complying with BA provisions

5. Confusion by individuals in understanding the NOPP (Most AHIMA Respondents Say HIPAA Uncovered "Problem Areas," 2004)

However, if failure to comply is found, then the following penalties may be imposed. A penalty of $100 per incidence may be imposed. Multiple violations in a calendar year may not exceed $25,000 per year. When the OCR finds a person knowingly obtained or disclosed PHI, a fine of $50,000 and imprisonment up to one year may be imposed. These criminal penalties may be increased to $100,000 and up to five years imprisonment if the wrongful conduct involves false pretenses, and up to $250,000 and ten years imprisonment if the conduct involves the intent to sell, transfer, or use IIHI for commercial advantage, personal gain, or malicious harm. These sanctions will be enforced by the Department of Justice. (OCR Privacy Rule Summary, 2003).

These penalties notwithstanding, it is the position of the DHHS that they strive to assist organizations to comply with the ruling. They do not want to prosecute. Their goal is to enable the system to work. As long as they find a willingness to adjust and correct situations, then enforcement is helpful, not something to fear.

Civil Penalties under HIPAA

Enough time has elapsed since HIPAA became enforceable law that court cases have begun to appear. Many health care providers and their staff are under the impression that they will be sued if they disclose PHI without proper authorization. Note the following scenario.

Chester Police Detective Sgt. Paul Willard of the Chester Pensylvania Police Department, "got a call from the nursing supervisor and she gave me holy hell. She asked me who I thought I was and said, 'You know, we could get sued.' I said I was just trying to conduct an investigation," recalled Willard. (Mengers, 2004).

Since patients have received their NOPP from health care providers, they have assumed a number of things that are not true about HIPAA. A misconception is that they have the option to sue the offending covered entity. The Fact Sheet from the DHHS's OCR states, "If you believe that a person, agency, or organization covered under the HIPAA Privacy Rule ("a covered entity") violated your (or someone else's) health information privacy rights or committed another violation of the Privacy Rule, you may file a complaint with the OCR." (OCR Fact Sheet, 2000). This clearly states that the only option is by means of complaint to the OCR.

Many grievances submitted to the Department of Justice have come under the category of plaintiffs suing for damages due to their PHI being used in ways claimed to be in violation of the HIPAA law. This is not permitted under HIPAA law. The only means for individuals to respond to unauthorized disclosure of their PHI is through filing a complaint with the OCR. Any petition submitted to the courts suing a covered entity for damages may be dismissed as inappropriate.

The memorandum from the Department of Justice (DOJ), Memorandum Opinion for The General Counsel Department of Health and Human Service and The Senior Counsel to the Deputy Attorney General, dated June 1, 2005, separates the civil penalties from the criminal penalties. Only a covered entity can be found guilty of civil violations when PHI is received or sent to another covered entity. An example given is "When using or disclosing PHI or when requesting PHI from another covered entity, the information requested should be limited to that which is *reasonably necessary*. Failure to comply with these regulations (minimum necessary) may render a covered entity either 'civilly or criminally liable' for obtaining individually identifiable health information in violation of the Privacy Rule." (Scope of Criminal Enforcement, 2005). The civil aspect of the ruling seems to focus on improper disclosure of IIHI or PHI more than is necessary or possibly without authorization.

Criminal Penalties under HIPAA

As of this writing, decisions in three prominent cases involving HIPAA enforcement have begun to establish precedence. Three criminal convictions have been handed down against individuals. The DOJ has carefully explained their definition of covered entities. Under the definition written in HIPAA law, a health care provider is a person furnishing health care services or supplies. This can be either an individual or an entity. The DOJ contrasts the definitions of health plan, health care clearinghouse, and prescription drug card sponsor by stating that they (covered entities) "will virtually never be an individual." (Scope of Criminal Enforcement, 2005). We refer to a Memorandum Opinion for The General Counsel, Department of Health and Human Services, and The Senior Counsel to the Deputy Attorney General, dated June 1, 2005. This opinion outlines the scope of criminal enforcement under the Administrative Simplification portion of HIPAA. It addresses the question of whether individual persons can be held liable or just the organizations defined as covered entities. If a covered entity is not an individual and it is found in violation of HIPAA regulations, it would fall under the corporate criminal liability category. The first criminal case was decided in August 2004. The plaintiff in the Western District of Washington pleaded guilty to "wrongful disclosure of individually identifiable health information for economic gain, a violation of 42 USC Section 1320d-6." In this case, the plaintiff used the information to obtain several credit cards. He was convicted as an individual since the DOJ has stated that the Privacy Rule can apply to members of a covered entity's workforce. The criminal provision makes it a crime to do certain acts knowingly and in violation of the Privacy Rule. (Scope of Criminal Enforcement, 2005). The opinion permits that a person, not a covered entity, would be capable of committing such an act. This validates the conviction of the gentleman who stole IIHI for economic gain.

The second criminal conviction occurred in Alamo, Texas, when a woman was convicted of selling medical records to an FBI agent (FBI Miami Field Division Press Release, 2006). The third conviction was announced in the Southern District of Florida. Two people were charged with various counts of conspiracy. One of the three counts was for violating HIPAA through the wrongful disclosure of IIHI. They used the stolen patient information to submit over $2 million in false claims to Medicare. (Southern District of Florida Press Release, 2006). Though disclosure of PHI may initiate an investigation from the OCR, there are real teeth in HIPAA law to bring both civil and criminal indictments against those who may use IIHI to their advantage.

The OCR has ten regional offices. Complaints are to be submitted to the appropriate regional office based on the region where the alleged violation took place. See the Appendix B for a listing of offices and a copy of the "Fact Sheet: How to File a Health Information Privacy Complaint," plus a copy of the downloadable complaint form. This is also available from the Web site http://www.hhs.gov. Search for "How to File a Health Information Privacy Complaint."

The memorandum opinion further explains when civil penalties and criminal penalties can be imposed. The secretary of DHHS may impose civil penalties on any person who violates a provision of HIPAA for not more than $100 for each violation. There are other limits if the violation is imposed on a covered entity as outlined previously.

The memorandum further describes that criminal sanctions can be imposed only for those violations of the standards that involve the disclosure of "unique health identifiers." "Any person(s) who knowingly uses or causes to be used a unique health identifier;

1. Obtains individually identifiable health information relating to an individual;

2. Discloses individually identifiable health information to another person, shall be punished as provided in…" the HIPAA Privacy Rule. (Scope of Criminal Enforcement, 2005).

What does this mean to the health care staff? It is vital to understand HIPAA limitations and provisions. No individual or staff member of a covered entity is exempt from review by the OCR if a complaint is leveled against their covered entity.

What the HIPAA Privacy Rule Covers

A report from the Delco Times states that law enforcement has frequently encountered problems frequently encountered problems with organizations overenthusiastic and apparently not well informed about HIPAA restrictions.

True Story

"A gentleman came to the (police) station for help. His wife was transported to the hospital for a psychiatric evaluation and she was transferred to another hospital and the hospital wouldn't tell him what hospital she was transferred to," said Pennsylvania State Police Sgt. Tony Sivo. "Public officials and public agencies often improperly cite HIPAA in denying access to information. In most cases they are not covered entities and are not covered by the provisions," per Teri Henning, media law counsel for the Pennsylvania Newspaper Association. (Mengers, 2004).

In the above scenario, the hospital had likely overreacted to the call for privacy of patient information. HIPAA allows discretion be used by the attending physician and staff to assist family members in caring for sick or injured family.

It has always been the case that appropriate court authority is required before health information can legitimately be released to law enforcement. HIPAA does not interfere with that longstanding situation. Court authority to release information trumps HIPAA and any health care provider's policy. HIPAA actually makes it easier for law enforcement to obtain information when there has been criminal activity associated with the health condition of a patient.

SUMMARY

The Privacy Rule written by the DHHS creates standards for protecting all IIHI in the country. Implementation began in April 2003 for all health care providers. It allows health care providers to access information to fully and adequately treat their patients. Each provider must have policies in place to comply with the Privacy Rule. The ruling allows each health care facility to comply in a manner that is "reasonable" for their particular setting.

The Privacy Rule applies to all covered entities. The focus is to ensure the privacy of PHI. Information is defined as PHI if a connection can be made between an individual and a health condition.

The Privacy Rule outlines when use or disclosure is permitted only with written authorization. Authorization may be granted to disclose PHI for a specific purpose. Authorization states what is to be disclosed, to whom it is to be disclosed, and when the authorization expires. There are exceptions dealing with parents and minor children. In any suspected case of domestic violence, abuse, or neglect, disclosure to authorities is mandatory.

Psychotherapy notes require specific authorization from the patient even if disclosure is for treatment, payment, or health care operations (TPO). All staff is to have access to the "minimum necessary" amount of PHI that is needed to fulfill their job responsibility. Clinical workers will have the greatest access since they treat the patient directly.

There are several permitted uses or disclosures of PHI without written authorization. These come under the category of "for the public interest or to benefit the public." Some PHI may be used for marketing purposes. The specifics are carefully outlined so individual health information is not distributed outside the scope of the covered entity solely for the purpose of selling a product or service. Patients, upon admission to an inpatient facility, have the choice to be listed in the published directory.

Many organizations work alongside health care providers who have access to some PHI as business associates. BAs agree to protect all health information they may encounter in their business dealings.

The Privacy Rule directed all providers to provide every patient with a Notice Of Privacy Practices. This outlines how PHI will be used and protected, and how the patient can contact the provider if there is a problem or complaint. Patients may amend their medical record if they disagree with its contents. Amendments are to be reviewed by the health care facility before being added to the record. This gives patients with false information in their record the opportunity to correct mistakes.

All health care workers are to receive HIPAA training when beginning their employment, with periodic retraining. When the OCR investigates complaints, HIPAA outlines when monetary penalties and criminal charges may be applied. If the OCR finds noncompliance and unwillingness toward compliance, they have the obligation to impose penalties in the form of fines. Criminal charges under HIPAA are reserved for persons who knowingly use IIHI for uses in violation of the HIPAA law.

REVIEW QUESTIONS

1. The receptionist for a physician is directed to call a patient with a reminder of an upcoming appointment. No one answers the phone, and she is directed to leave a voice message; what can be said? The same "how to do it" question comes up with mailing appointment reminders. Are these postcard reminders illegal under HIPAA law?

2. To prevent patients from overhearing discussions with the doctor, must all examining rooms be soundproofed?

3. A hospital uses protected health information (PHI) about an individual to provide health care to the individual and consults with other health care providers about the individual's treatment. Is authorization needed?

4. A psychoanalyst forwards a patient's health care information to another health care provider for further treatment by that provider. Is authorization needed?

5. A hospital sends a patient's health care instructions to a nursing home to which the patient is being transferred. Is authorization needed?

6. A contract computer repairperson asks for the logon and password to test a computer. She has signed a business associate contract; can she have access?

7. Marketing scenarios:

   a) An advertisement is received from a hospital informing former patients about a cardiac facility, which is not part of the hospital, that can provide a baseline EKG for $39. The communication is not for the purpose of providing treatment advice. Is this considered marketing?

   b) A hospital uses its patient list to announce the arrival of a new specialty group (e.g., orthopedic) or the acquisition of new equipment (e.g., X-ray machine) through a general mailing or publication. Is this considered marketing?

c) A primary care physician refers an individual to a specialist for a follow-up test or provides free samples of a prescription drug to a patient. Is this considered marketing?

d) A hospital provides a free package of formula and other baby products to new mothers as they leave the maternity ward. Is this considered marketing?

8. What does the term "covered entity" mean? What are the three categories of covered entities? Discuss some of the varieties of covered entities that must be compliant with HIPAA and some that might not be covered entities.

9. Authorizations generally give permission for a specific time limit. Why does this protect privacy?

10. The Privacy Rule allows patients to see a list of disclosures of their PHI. This excludes those disclosures for TPO. What other disclosures would be possible?

11. Why is it important that the HIPAA Privacy Rule cover business associates?

REFERENCES

Black Eye at the Med Center. (1999, February 22). *Washington Business.*

California appellate court says plaintiff's signed release bars HIV privacy suit. (2000, February 22). *AIDS Litigation Reporter.*

Crowley, S. (2000, March). Invading Your Medical Privacy. *AARP Bulletin,* p. 1.

Duke, Nicole H. (2006). First Criminal Case Conviction Under HIPAA, *VP Publications Kaufman & Canoles.* Retrieved January 19, 2007, from http://www.kaufcan.com/pubTemplates/articles.asp?

Hillig, T. and Mannies, J. (2001, July 3). Woman sues over posting of abortion details. *St. Louis Post-Dispatch*, p. A1.

HIPAA Electronic Transaction and Code Sets. (March 2003). Volume 1, Paper 1, Centers for Medicare and Medicaid Services, p. 1.

HIPAA Readiness Checklist. (2003, March). Centers for Medicare and Medicaid Services. p. 1.

Mengers, P. (2004, May 2). The HIPAA effect: Privacy matters. *Delco Times.* Retrieved January 17, 2007, from http://www.zwire.com/site/index.cfm.

Most AHIMA Survey Respondents Say HIPAA Uncovered "Problem Areas," *Report on Patient Privacy.* (May 2004). Atlantic Information Service, Inc., p. 3.

OCR Fact Sheet (June 2000). p. 1. Retrieved January 19, 2007, from http://www.hhs.gov/ocr/privacyhowtofile.htm.

OCR Privacy Rule Summary. (April 2003). Summary of the HIPAA Privacy Rule, p. 4.

Personal Representatives OCR HIPAA Privacy (2002, December 3, revised April 3, 2003) (codified at 45 C.F.R.164.502(g)). p. 1. Retrieved January 15, 2007, from http://www.hhs.gov/ocr/hipaa/guidelines/personalrepresentative.pdf.

Psychotherapy Notes, Standards for Privacy of Individually Identifiable Health Information No. 250, 65 Fed. Reg. 82,622–82, 623. (December 28, 2000).

Requirements for Policies and Procedures, and Documentation Requirements, 65 Fed Reg. 82,563 (December 28, 2000).

Scope of Criminal Enforcement Under 42 USC Section 132d-6, June 1, 2005, p 6. Department of Justice. Retrieved January 27, 2007, from http://www.usdoj.gov/olc/hipaa_final.htm (pg 3/12 memorandum opinion of DOJ, June 2005).

Southern District of Florida Press Release. Two charges in computer fraud, identity theft and health care fraud conspiracy. (September 8, 2006). Retrieved January 12, 2007, from http://www.usdoj.gov.

Standards for Privacy of Individually Identifiable Health Information; Final Rule, 67 Fed. Reg. 53,182–53,215 (2002, August 14).

Stein, R. (2006, June 5). Enforcement of HIPAA draws mixed reviews. *Fort Worth Star-Telegram (TX)*, NewsBank, p. A6. Retrieved January 19, 2007 from http://infoweb.newsbank.com.

Two charged in computer fraud, identity theft and health care fraud conspiracy, FBI Miami Field Division Press 1Release. (September 6, 2005). Retrieved January 12, 2007, from http://www.usdoj.gov/usaofls/PressReleases.

Woman faces prison for attempted sale of FBI medical records. (March 20, 2006.) FBI Miami Field Division Press Release. Retrieved January 19, 2007, from http://www.itcinstitute.com/print/aspx.

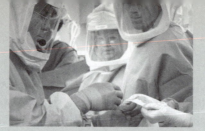

CHAPTER

3

TRANSACTIONS AND CODE SETS

OBJECTIVES

Explain the need for national standards for electronic transactions.

Identify the code sets mandated by HIPAA law.

Explain the structure of the electronic transactions to simplify reimbursement for health care services.

Recognize the value of trading partner agreements.

Understand the enforcement guidelines set up by the Department of Health and Human Services.

KEY TERMS

adjudication
ASC X12 standards
biologic
code set
crossover claim
electronic data
   interchange (EDI)
etiology
Explanation of Benefits
   (EOB)

format
HCPCS—Health [Care
   Financing
   Administration]
   Common Procedure
   Coding System
nomenclatures
Office of E-Health
   Standards and
   Services (OESS)

Office of HIPAA
   Standards (OHS)
orthotic
protocol
provider taxonomy code
subscriber
trading partner
trading partner
   agreement (TPA)
X12N

INTRODUCTION

*A**nother federal mandate affecting the flow of health care information takes the form of consistently formatting transmissions of electronic protected health information (e-PHI). In order for all parties to communicate efficiently, a standard must be defined so each health plan, health care provider, and health care clearinghouse can communicate with each other. In other words, all parties must adopt a common language. The Department of Health and Human Services (DHHS) looked to the standards in the business world and found that the Accredited Standards Committee (ASC) had developed standards that have been tested and found secure and efficient for most other industries. The next step was to define the language to use in electronic health care transactions and the form or architecture of these transactions. The Standards for Electronic Transactions were finalized in October 2000. A Final Rule titled Modifications to Electronic Data Transaction Standards and Code Sets was printed in the Federal Register in February 2003. Small health plans were permitted a final date of October 2004. Any transaction of e-PHI between any of the three covered entities must be translated or formatted into the federal standard. This was good news for the health care provider since the abundant varieties of claim forms disappeared. It also brought a problem for the health plans that wanted certain other types of information to better **adjudicate**, or process, their claims. Explanation of the various parts of this ruling follows.*

THINK ABOUT IT

1. Computer code is like a foreign language. Do I need to learn this language to understand electronic date interchange (EDI) transactions?
2. If a facility sends all claims to a clearinghouse, is it important for the provider to understand transaction details?
3. What is the cost in staff-hours to the health care provider if a claim needs to be resubmitted?
4. How can HIPAA compliance lessen the need to resubmit claims?

Purpose of Transaction Standards

The Transaction and Code Sets portion of HIPAA Administrative Simplification is the heart of where the promised savings and simplification are realized. With implementation of this section of the Health Insurance Portability and Accountability Act, health care providers begin to see that accounts receivable days shrink, increasing the cash flow to their organization. The cost of office overhead shrinks also. Patients know at the time of their visit the exact insurance coverage they are able to receive. All this elevates the level of confidence conveyed to patients in a health care facility.

The health care industry was the only major industry in the United States that processed the majority of its transactions on paper. It did not seriously consider standardizing transactions even on paper. Banks, money exchanges, stock exchanges, steel plants, manufacturing plants, and many others conducted business in a secure electronic **format** based on **electronic data interchange (EDI)**. An electronic format is an arrangement of data elements that assist in identifying the contents of a transaction. Since the use of EDI began, many businesses have streamlined manual and tedious data entry tasks. The overall expense of doing business has shrunk for organizations of all sizes. Congress motivated the health care providers to use a tried-and-true process.

The administrative simplification provisions of HIPAA law were passed with the support of the health care industry. Only with federal government help would all individual providers be able to submit transactions in a uniform way. Individual health plans could not agree on a standard without giving competitors a market advantage. The HIPAA law levels the playing field for all health plans. It does not require all transactions be submitted electronically, but those that are submitted in that manner are now standardized. (Department of Health and Human Services, 2003).

The ASC has developed standards for cross-industry exchange of electronic business information since the 1980s. By the year 2000, more than 300,000 companies had used EDI and the ASC X12 system to transmit information. This electronic system is defined as computer-to-computer transmission of business information in a standard format using national standard communications **protocols**, or a set of conventions, governing the formatting of data in an electronic communications system. By using this electronic interchange with their business partners, industries have saved billions of dollars in office costs. Businesses have greatly expanded the reach of their markets through this secure and streamlined exchange of data. Note the remarkable efficiencies used extensively in the auto industry that make "just-in-time" processes work.

Inventory is tracked in detail so a minimum of warehouse space is used to store parts.

Prior to HIPAA there were more than 300 standards for electronic transactions. The ASC now oversees the development of all standards. Changes are implemented only after a consensus of those using standards. This has benefited the non-health care business world for over 25 years. Businesses have seen reduced cycle time of their inventory, increased productivity, reduced costs, improved accuracy, improved business relationships, enhanced customer service, increased sales, minimized paper use and storage, and increased cash flow. Certainly there are similar benefits to the health care industry as they use **ASC X12 standards**.

EDI allows offices to transmit and receive information without rekeying or other human intervention. Information contained in an EDI transaction set is, for the most part, the same as on conventional documents. The impact to the health care provider and payer is that information will be transmitted via instantaneous electronic means rather than slow-moving paper. The same information required for a paper insurance claim is still needed. The electronic transmission is immensely efficient and time saving. The challenge for the covered entities is to manage the hardware and software that transmits this information. A typical medical office assistant, doctor, or clinical worker needs to understand the workings of the transaction. They need to understand who can train them and who can assist when errors occur. HIPAA has initially adopted eight standards for use with transmitting e-PHI, and there are more standards being considered for adoption. The DHHS has not finalized a *claims attachment* format as of 2007.

Parts 160 and 162 of Title II in the HIPAA statute outlines standards for eight approved electronic transactions and for the code sets to be used in those transactions. These eight original forms for electronic communication are to be used exclusively between health plans, health care clearinghouses, and health care providers. This Transaction and Code Sets Rule does not eliminate the use of paper claims submitted on CMS-1500, UB-04, or dental forms. These are still permitted and in some limited cases preferable. In time, even the paper exceptions will be phased out in favor of the electronic medical records (EMR). Claims where the charges require explanation still need to be submitted on paper with supporting documentation until the standard for attachments to health claims has been implemented. The planning committees are developing some means of explanation to be included within the transaction set so the need for supporting documentation will be reduced even further. The rule addresses the use of electronic media to transmit e-PHI between health plans, health care clearinghouses, and certain health care providers. The definition of "certain health care providers" includes only those who transmit any health information in electronic form in connection with a transaction covered by this portion of HIPAA. The ruling applies only when the health care provider transmits claims electronically.

Each covered entity needs to manage the transmission of health care information in accordance with the Transaction and Code Sets Rule. This means that all covered entities such as all private health plans, including managed care programs, and government health plans such as Medicare, state Medicaid programs, the military health care system, the Veterans Health Administration, and Indian Health Service programs will send and receive standard transactions. Any health care clearinghouse is also a covered entity.

The term "covered entity" is limited to providers who transmit any health information in electronic form in connection with a HIPAA standard transaction. The Administrative Simplification Compliance Act Enforcement of Mandatory Electronic Submission of Medicare Claims has a list of eight exceptions to the health care providers who are covered entities. They are as follows:

1. A small provider—a provider billing a Medicare fiscal intermediary that has fewer than 25 full-time equivalent employees (FTEs), and a physician, practitioner, or supplier with fewer than 10 FTEs that bills a Medicare carrier

2. A dentist

3. A participant in a Medicare demonstration project in which paper claim filing is required due to the inability of the applicable *Implementation Guide,* adopted under HIPAA, to report data essential for the demonstration

4. A provider that conducts mass immunizations, such as flu injections; they may be permitted to submit paper roster bills

5. A provider that submits claims when more than one other payer is responsible for payment prior to Medicare payment

6. A provider that only furnishes services outside of the United States

7. A provider experiencing a disruption in electricity and communication connections that is beyond its control

8. A provider who can establish that an "unusual circumstance" exists that precluded submission of claims electronically. (ASCA Enforcement, 2005)

In this article, which had an effective date of July 2005, any other health care provider, i.e., a covered entity, is advised that Medicare payments will be affected. The federal government is moving to mandate that all providers submit claims electronically. Just because a provider is a listed exception does not give an excuse to dismiss these rules. The HIPAA officer needs to look to the future and move towards electronic claims submission.

There is a certain amount of information one needs to know before one can manage EDI. It is not necessary to be an expert in electronic transmissions. It is like knowing and using electricity. Most of us understand some basic elements of electricity, yet the complete knowledge of exactly how it works is not necessary to use electricity effectively. A trusted software vendor should be retained who is qualified to implement and support EDI applications. The workforce must have enough understanding to know when to call for outside help. Training should focus on accurate and acceptable transmissions. Questions should first be asked of the software vendor. The Centers for Medicare and Medicaid Services (CMS), who oversee compliance, are another source for help. There should be training for certain individuals within the organization to operate the software and hardware to make the transmissions secure.

Submitting paper claims is a poor option since it continues to be costly. One of the disadvantages is that it extends the accounts payable time to collect the money due the health care provider. The cost of following up with phone calls, printing and mailing billing statements, and eventually having a collection agency contact the insured reduces the actual funds the physician receives for patient care. Bad debt increases sharply on aging accounts. The initial cost of transition to electronic claim submission means an investment of computer equipment and software to be able to handle the change. Software vendors will adjust their products as the processes are changed. We have seen the inevitable change to EDI become acceptable, desired, and pervasive.

DESIGNATED CODE SETS

EDI requires certain coding to explain lengthy descriptions. Under HIPAA, a **code set** is any set of codes used for encoding data elements, such as tables of terms, medical concepts, medical diagnosis, or medical procedure. The medical and clinical codes explain the diagnosis, procedure performed, drug used, services rendered, and supplies provided. It standardizes the codes to be used and eliminates local and health plan issued codes. The Transaction and Code Sets Rule designates certain sources to be used to code items such as diagnoses, procedures for outpatients and inpatients, drugs and biologics, and dental procedures. Medicare originated a **Health Care [Financing Administration] Procedure Coding System (HCPCS)**, nicknamed "hick-pick," which lists codes that are referred to as Level II codes. Medicare has endorsed the CPT-4 coding and the HCPCS and often refers to these two systems of procedural codes as HCPCS Level I and Level II codes. Level III codes have been eliminated due to HIPAA law. The other category of codes is nonmedical codes. Some examples are state abbreviations, provider specialty, and remittance remarks to explain adjustments on a remittance. In a response to a claim, there are several categories of codes used to codify reasons relating to the judgment for or against payment or adjudication of the claim. Medical codes pertain to a patient encounter.

Diagnosis Codes

The International Classification of Diseases, 9th edition, Clinical Modification, (ICD-9-CM) Volumes 1 and 2 are to be used to report only diagnoses. These include diseases, injuries, medical conditions, and other health-related problems and their manifestations. This reference book, ICD-9-CM, as a printed text is updated yearly. Since 2005, the DHHS has issued revisions twice a year on April 1 and October 1. The revised codes are available on the Centers for Disease Control and Prevention Web site, http://www.cdc.gov. Search for National Center for Health Statistics, "disease classification." This change is a result of the Medicare Prescription Drug, Improvement, and Modernization Act of 2003.

The field of mental health relies on the *Diagnostic and Statistical Manual of Mental Disorders*, 4th edition, Text Revision (DSM-IV-TR) for diagnostic codes. This reference was not part of the code sets adopted by the DHHS for inclusion on EDI. Any mental disorders must be identified using the ICD-9-CM code set. In some cases the DSM-IV-TR codes include greater diagnostic specificity than ICD-9-CM. Because of that, new codes have been added to the ICD-9-CM text to accommodate these distinctions. Mental health facilities are not prohibited from using the DSM-IV-TR in their practice but must convert the codes and descriptors to adopted code sets when entering them on electronic standard transactions. (DSM-IV-TR, 2006)

It is important to note that the World Health Organization (WHO) revises the *International Classification of Diseases*. The tenth revision has the support of the National Center for Health Statistics, CMS, and the American Health Information Management Association (AHIMA).The clinical modifications have been complete for several years. The change to the ICD-10-CM diagnosis coding will be one of the next issues facing the health care industry. This coding system for diagnoses and injuries will increase the coding system to six spaces with both alpha and numeric identifiers. The tenth revision includes laterality—which side—within the code itself. Many new understandings of disease and the **etiology** (all causes of a disease or abnormal condition) of conditions have changed since 1975, when the ninth classification of diseases was developed. As a result, the tenth revision groups some diseases differently from the ninth revision.

Inpatient Procedure Codes

Procedures for diseases, injuries, and medical complications performed on inpatients are to be coded from Volume 3 of ICD-9-CM. This does not change inpatient coding from the prior standard. This volume is used only by hospitals, long-term care facilities, and similar inpatient institutions, and for claims on inpatients.

These four-digit codes are currently being used by hospitals to report prevention, diagnosis, treatment, and management procedures. This volume is updated yearly, and new codes are valid beginning January 1 of each year. Many publishers provide all three volumes of the ICD-9-CM in one text. Many software vendors provide programs for coding that are based on the ICD-9-CM. The software, called an encoder, asks a series of questions to establish an appropriate coding path. This helps the coder to find the correct code by eliminating all other options.

Just as there has been a move by organizations like AHIMA and others to incorporate the ICD-10-CM diagnosis coding into the United States standards, there is also a similar move to adopt procedural coding of the International Classification of Diseases,10th Revision Procedure Coding System (ICD-10-PCS). The CMS arranged with 3-M Health Information Systems to develop a more comprehensive system of procedural coding to replace the ICD-9-CM procedure codes. The ICD-10-PCS has been developed to complement the diagnosis system. It is designed in a very different manner from the current CPT-4 coding system or the Volume 3 ICD-9-CM procedures. There are a total of seven characters for each procedure listed. By using both letters and numbers, there are a possible 34 different values for each of the seven spaces. The letters "O" and "I" are not used so there is no confusion with the numbers zero (0) and one (1). This system of coding does not include any diagnostic information, only a procedure and its method of delivery (how it was accomplished).

Outpatient Procedure Codes

Procedure codes for *physician services* and other health-related services are found in the *Current Procedural Terminology,* 4th edition (CPT-4) This is the HCPCS Level I coding system. The American Medical Association (AMA) maintains this coding system. These codes are five digits without any decimal. They include evaluation and management (E/M) services, anesthesia procedures, surgical procedures, radiology, pathology and laboratory services, as well as services dealing with medicines and their application to the patient. This last section includes psychiatry procedures, ophthalmology procedures, therapeutic cardiovascular services, and therapies of various types among other services. New codes are released twice yearly—January 1 and July 1 of each year—and are valid six months after released. These new codes may be accessed from the AMA Web site.

The Healthcare Common Procedural Coding System (HCPCS Level II) contains codes for physician services as well as many other *nonphysician provided health care services and equipment*. The HCPCS Level II codes are updated annually with new codes being valid January 1 each year and distributed by the DHHS. If services and provisions are *not administered by a physician*, then HCPCS is the place to find that alphanumeric code. The HCPCS codes list substances, equipment, supplies, and other items used in health care services. This may include items like ambulance and other transporting services, medical supplies, **orthotic** (a support or brace for weak or ineffective joints or muscles) and prosthetic devices, and durable medical equipment. These codes consist of six characters. The first is a letter followed by five digits. Level III codes, which were state- or health plan–specific, were eliminated in favor of standardization.

The AMA has worked on improving the structure and process of *Current Procedural Terminology*, 4th edition (CPT-4). These procedures are to include both inpatient and outpatient procedural coding. Changes in this system, *Current Procedural Terminology*, 5th edition (CPT-5), will be only minor and generally will include revised and new codes. It is anticipated that when there is the move to ICD-10 version coding, the CPT-5 will also be implemented.

Dental Procedures

Dentists use a separate coding book referred to as *Current Dental Terminology*, version 4. This is commonly referred to as CDT-4, an American Dental Association (ADA) publication. These are revised biannually starting January 1 of odd-numbered years—2005, 2007, and 2009, for example. These codes are a subset of Common Procedure Coding System (HCPCS Level II) codes since they begin with the letter "D" followed by four digits.

Drug Codes

The DHHS designated that drugs are to be coded from the National Drug Code (NDC) System. This listing of drugs was established under the Medicare program. The National Drug Code serves as a universal product identifier for drug reimbursement for retail pharmacy drug transactions. It is updated by the DHHS in collaboration with drug manufacturers. These codes are to be used by retail pharmacies to list drugs used to fill doctors' prescriptions. This includes both drugs and **biologics**. Biologics are products that are used to make medicines. The codes are unique 10-digit, three-segment numbers. Each number identifies the labeler, vendor, product, and trade package size. The NDC uses one of the following configurations: 4-4-2, 5-3-2, or 5-4-1. The first segment of the identifier indicates the firm that manufacturers, repackages, or distributes a drug product. The drug manufacturer assigns the product and package numbers—the second and third portions of the code. Drugs listed in the NDC are limited to prescription drugs and a few selected over-the-counter (OTC) products. Details about any drug can be found at the Web site for the United States Food and Drug Administration, http://www.fda.gov.

Nonmedical Code Sets

HIPAA defined nonmedical code sets strictly for administrative purposes. These codes do not refer directly to the medical care of a patient. They include items in an insurance claim such as state abbreviations, zip codes, telephone area codes, race, and ethnicity codes. There are code sets developed for use in the electronic transaction to identify the physician's specialty training, payment policies, the status of a claim and why claims have been denied or adjusted, type of health plan, benefits and patient eligibility, provider organization type, disability type, and reasons for rejection, to name a few.

In order to identify the specialty training for a particular doctor, there is a **provider taxonomy code**. The National Uniform Claim Committee (NUCC) Data Subcommittee maintains this set of codes. These codes identify the provider type and area(s) of specialization for each health care provider. The new coding system is to be free from identifiers so that the location or specialty of the physician cannot be determined. Use of the taxonomy code will enable health care providers to identify their specialty field to a health plan.

There are several other code sets that help explain decisions of the health plan. Other sets of these nonmedical codes are *claim adjustment reason codes* and *reject reason codes*. These codes explain the payment policies that affect reimbursement. These standardized codes eliminate the need for **Explanation of Benefits (EOB)** sent to the provider explaining the reasons for adjusted payment by service line.

Another type of code is *remittance advance remark codes*. When information is lacking or needs further clarification, one of these codes is returned to the provider for clarification of the rejection.

Claim status codes and *claim status category codes* communicate to the health care provider a particular claim's status. The category code of "F2" means the claim or line has been denied. Other codes explain detail about the status, such as entity is not approved as an electronic submitter, special handling required at health plan site, or duplicate of a previously processed claim or line. These are examples of nonmedical code sets that the Department of Health and Human Services has adopted for the EDI transmissions.

ASC X12 NOMENCLATURE

The American National Standards Institute (ANSI) is recognized in the world as an authoritative organization to set standards. This organization is given the authority to develop standards and give them **nomenclatures**, meaning names, that are recognized internationally. The Accredited Standards Committee (ASC) and the DHHS created a new committee—National Uniform Claim Committee (NUCC)—to develop a standardized data set to be implemented for HIPAA transactions formerly sent on the CMS-1500 form. The National Uniform Claim Committee (NUCC) sets the standards for content and data definitions for noninstitutional health care claims in the United States. The standardized data set outlines how and in what order the information is to be sent through EDI in the ASC **X12N** standard to and from third-party payers. The "X12 N" nomenclature designates the EDI standards for the Insurance Industry. The NUCC consists of representatives from the AMA, CMS, key provider and payer organizations, and state and federal regulators. There was representation from both health care providers and health care payers. Their recommendations complement the work of the Accredited Standards Committee on Electronic Date Interchange (ASC X12N) to comply with the HIPAA law.

Washington Publishing Company (WPC) has developed implementation guides for assisting information management technicians to administer and support the X12N transmissions. The "N" transmissions are the transaction standards for the insurance industry. The WPC manages the manufacturing and distribution process and holds the copyright for the X12N implementation guides on behalf of the X12N Subcommittee.

DATA OVERVIEW

To understand a little of what is going through the communication wires in EDI, we will examine some of the terms and ideas of computer communications. Any one transaction set contains groups of logically related data in units called segments. A data element is the smallest named unit of information in the ASC X12 standard. For instance, the "N4" segment used in the transaction set conveys the city, state, zip code, and other geographic information. A transaction set contains multiple segments, so the addresses of the different parties, for example, can be conveyed from one computer to the other. An analogy would be that the transaction set is like a freight train: the segments are like the train's cars and each segment can contain several data elements in the same manner that a train car can hold multiple crates. (ACS X12N Guide, 2000). The information is sent with a "header" and a "trailer" segment. These tell the computer when to start and end the "claim." These markers define the data element separators and terminator. They identify the sender and receiver. The markers provide controls for the interchange and also allow authorization and security for the transmission.

Architecture

The ASC has set up templates, meaning the architecture, for each of their defined transactions. The WPC in Rockville, Maryland, is responsible for maintaining and providing Internet access to these standards. Their Web site is http://www.wpc-edi.com. The transactions created in the Transaction and Code Sets Rule are the following:

1. ASC X12N 837—Health Care Claim: Dental, Professional, or Institutional

2. ASC X12N 270—Health Care Eligibility Benefit Inquiry

3. ASC X12N 271—Health Care Eligibility Benefit Response

4. ASC X12N 276—Health Care Claim Status Request

5. ASC X12N 277—Health Care Claim Status Response

6. ASC X12N 278—Health Care Services Review

7. ASC X12N 834—Benefit Enrollment and Maintenance

8. ASC X12N 835—Health Care Claim Payment/Advise

The transaction templates are the first ones accepted by the federal government to send and receive e-PHI between providers and payers. Health care personnel do need to understand the details of these transactions. Since HIPAA does not specify how the provider complies, software vendors have provided many options for health care providers to use. The health care provider is responsible for being certain that the formats they use comply with the HIPAA standards. The software vendor is performing a service to the provider to make life easier. The ultimate responsibility for accuracy lies with the provider.

The following titles are for claim forms:

Health Care Institutional ASC X12N 837, version 4010 X 96

Health Care Dental ASC X12N 837, version 4010 X 097

Health Care Professional ASC X12N 837, version 4010 X 98

There are three versions of the claim form, which cover institutional and hospital claims, dental claims, and physician claims. The paper forms for dentists, doctors, and hospitals have been different so the electronic format is unique to accommodate these differences. The institutional claim covers hospitals, nursing facilities, and similar inpatient institutions. The professional version is designed for physician services as well as providers of durable medical equipment and similar suppliers. In time, as needs change, these transaction standards have a lot of flexibility to adapt easily in the future. We will look at a sample of an institutional form.

Health Care Eligibility Benefit Inquiry ASC X12N 270 is used to inquire concerning a patient's eligibility for benefits from a health plan or to determine if a specific procedure is covered (eligible for payment) under the patient's policy. The companion form Health Care Eligibility Benefit Response ASC X12N 271 is the standard for reply. The efficiency of an electronic request and almost immediate reply provides more time to take care of the patient needs in a timely manner. This also permits physicians to discuss options at the time of treatment with the patient if coverage is denied or only partially covered.

Health Care Claim Status Request ASC X12N 276 requests information about the status of the claim that has been transmitted. The reply uses Health Care Claim Response ASC X12N 277 format. A typical code reply may be "P3"—pending or requesting information, "F2"—finalized or denied, or "R3"—requests for additional information, or another claim, or another line on the claim.

Health Care Services Review ASC X12N 278 is the standard for electronic exchange of requests and responses between health care providers and health plans in regard to certification and authorization for procedures. It is standard to receive an authorization number from a health plan and include that number on the claim form. This helps assure that services will be paid. It can also provide information to the health care provider regarding how much the plan will pay for specific procedures. This information allows the physician to better assess the means to treat the patient in question and to advise them of what to expect from their health plan. With a secondary and possibly a tertiary payer, this request allows the provider to quickly receive information from all parties involved in payment.

The form Health Care Services Review/Request X12N 278 allows authorization for a patient to be referred to another provider. With many preferred provider organizations (PPO), the options for referrals are limited to a specific list. The primary physician is able quickly to determine if a provider is authorized.

Benefit Enrollment and Maintenance ASC X12N 834 enables health care providers and health plans to exchange individual, **subscriber** (person named as the holder of the insurance policy), and dependent enrollment information. As policies change for particular plans, the health care provider can keep abreast of any changes of the policy. The extent of e-PHI that can be included in this transaction is limited to the "minimum necessary" for proper response. A health care provider will also be able to receive information concerning "disenrollment" from a health plan. By not paying premiums, a patient may be disenrolled from the health plan or may change employment and not continue the same coverage. Medicaid provisions are reviewed monthly by each state agency so eligibility for aid may change on a monthly basis. It is important to request current status so payment for services can be requested from the patient or guarantor if coverage is suspended or cancelled.

Health Care Claim Payment Advice ASC X12N 835 is the transaction coming from the health plan with remittance advice, much the same as the Coordination of Benefits. The transmission includes two pieces of information: the payment with information about the transfer of funds and the explanation of benefits detailing coverage of billed procedures and services. With electronic banking, providers can receive payments to their bank accounts via electronic transfer. This puts funds into the health care provider's available cash flow almost immediately after services are provided. The explanation of benefits portion of the reply advises the health care provider of any adjustments, deductible amounts for the guarantor to pay, and other pertinent information about payment of the claim.

Additional Information to Support a Health Care Claim or Encounter Transaction ASC X12N 275 is proposed for adoption for certain attachments to original claim. Use of this standard transaction would be to request further information about items such as laboratory results, emergency department services, ambulance services, medications, clinical reports, and nine rehabilitation specialties. It is not to include any information already sent in the claim transaction. The health plan would send a request via X12N 277. The provider would use the form X12N 275, Additional Information Request, for their reply. Since the inception of HIPAA transactions, health plans have begun to limit their requests to specific information rather than physician reports or notes. The use of this format is in keeping with the Privacy Rule policy of only disclosing the "minimum necessary" to accomplish the intended purpose of the request. To date, this has been used as a test program only. (HIPAA Administrative Simplification, 2005).

Table 3-1 lists transactions covered by HIPAA.

TABLE 3-1 Transactions Covered by HIPPA

ASC X12N	Title	Function	Prior Form
837: Version 4010 ×96	Health Care Claim: Dental	Bill for dental services	CMS-1500
837: Version 4010 ×97	Health Care Claim: Professional	Bill for physician and non-physician provided services or goods	CMS-1500
837: Version 4010 ×98	Health Care Claim: Institutional	Bill for institutional services: hospitals, nursing facilities, inpatient facilities	UB-04
270	Health Care Eligibility Benefit Inquiry	Request if specific procedure is eligible for payment	None
271	Health Care Eligibility Benefit Response	Reply from health plan re: payment for procedure	None
276	Health Care Claim Status Request	Request reply re: status of claim submitted but not paid	None
277	Health Care Claim Status Response	Reply from health plan re: why they are holding claim if received	None
278	Health Care Services Review	Health plan authorizes referral to another provider	None
834	Benefit Enrollment and Maintenance	Request and reply to determine if patient is enrolled in benefit plan.	None
835	Health Care Claim Payment/Advice	Remittance advice from health plan including electronic transfer of funds information	None
275: Proposed rule as of 2007	Additional Information request	Request for additional information from provider needed to adjudicate claim	None

Use of Loops

The architecture of the file is set up with many different loops. Loops are parts of information taken from the insurance claim form, either CMS-1500 for physician and supplier services, or UB-04 in the case of inpatient billing. Each loop contains a piece of information needed to complete the claim. As with paper insurance forms, there are more options or loops than needed every time. Only the loop that has information populated in it is sent as the data string. The first section is the header. This begins the data string and identifies the "engine," the type of transaction, who is submitting the claim, and who is to receive the claim. The next category gives detailed information about the billing party and information about electronic debiting of the account so payment can be made electronically. Then information about the subscriber or insured is transmitted. Other loops include the patient name and demographic information. The largest loop is the claim detail information. This includes dates of admission to the hospital, if applicable, the amount patient has paid on account, and all identification needed for authorization or referral. The diagnosis information, procedures performed, and their charges are listed in this loop. Other loops (when applicable) include information about the attending physician, operating physician, service facility, and other payer information when a secondary insurance is available. Finally is the "caboose" data, which tells the computer the end of the claim has been reached.

We will look at the information from a sample insurance claim that would be sent by a hospital for a patient who is the same as the subscriber. See Figure 3-1 for a sample UB-04 claim form. The two charges included are for preliminary blood test, CPT code: 85025—Hemogram and platelet count, automated, and automated partial differential WBC count, and CPT code: 93005—Electrocardiogram, tracing only without interpretation. These are procedures in preparation for cataract surgery. Principal diagnosis is 366.9: Unspecified cataract. Secondary diagnoses are 401.9: Unspecified essential hypertension and 794.31: Abnormal electrocardiogram. The inpatient surgery is ICD-9-CM, Vol. 3 procedure 15.3: Operations on two or more extraocular muscles involving temporary detachment from globe, one or both eyes. Here is the information in the traditional UB-04 format on paper. Following is the listing of information included in the data string for the electronic transmission.

Sample of EDI Claim Data (UB-04, Hospital Billing Form)

ASC X12N 837 Institutional Health Care Claim

Business Scenario—837 Institutional Claim

Patient is the same person as the Subscriber. The Primary Payer is Medicare and the Secondary payer is State Teachers. The Bill is a 141 Type of Bill (Medicare patient coming to the hospital for referenced diagnostic services).

Primary Payer Subscriber: John T Doe
Subscriber Address: 125 City Avenue Centerville PA 17111
Sex: M
DOB: 11/11/1936
Medicare insurance ID#: 030005074A
Payer ID #: 00435
Patient: Same as Primary Subscriber
Destination Payer: Medicare B
Submitter: Jones Hospital
EDI# 12345
Receiver: Medicare

1 BARKLEY BUILDING	2		3a PAT. CNTL # 7560480		4 TYPE OF BILL
JONES HOSPITAL			b. MED. REC. #		141
225 MAIN STREET		5 FED. TAX NO.	6 STATEMENT COVERS PERIOD FROM / THROUGH	7	
CENTERVILLE PA 17111			09112007 / 09112007		

8 PATIENT NAME	a DOE JOHN T	9 PATIENT ADDRESS	a 125 CITY AVENUE CENTERVILLE PA 17111
b		b	c / d / e

10 BIRTHDATE	11 SEX	12 DATE	13 HR	14 TYPE	15 SRC	16 DHR	17 STAT	18 19 20 21 CONDITION CODES 22 23 24 25 26 27 28	29 ACDT STATE	30
11111936	M	09112007		1			09			

31 OCCURRENCE CODE DATE	32 OCCURRENCE CODE DATE	33 OCCURRENCE CODE DATE	34 OCCURRENCE CODE DATE	35 OCCURRENCE SPAN CODE FROM THROUGH	36 OCCURRENCE SPAN CODE FROM THROUGH	37
A1 11111936	A2 11011991	B1 11111936	B2 01011987			

38 DOE JOHN T		39 CODE VALUE CODES AMOUNT	40 CODE VALUE CODES AMOUNT	41 CODE VALUE CODES AMOUNT
125 CITY AVENUE		a A2 15 31		
CENTERVILLE PA 17111		b		
		c		
		d		

42 REV. CD.	43 DESCRIPTION	44 HCPCS / RATE / HIPPS CODE	45 SERV. DATE	46 SERV. UNITS	47 TOTAL CHARGES	48 NON-COVERED CHARGES	49
1 305		85025		1	13 39		1
2 730		93005		1	76 54		2
3							3
4 001					89 93		4

PAGE 1 OF 1	CREATION DATE 09152007	TOTALS →	89 93

50 PAYER NAME	51 HEALTH PLAN ID	52 REL INFO	53 ASG BEN.	54 PRIOR PAYMENTS	55 EST. AMOUNT DUE	56 NPI
A MEDICARE	330127	Y	Y		89 93	57
B STATE TEACHERS	1135					OTHER PRV ID
C						

58 INSURED'S NAME	59 P.REL	60 INSURED'S UNIQUE ID	61 GROUP NAME	62 INSURANCE GROUP NO.
A DOE JOHN T	01	030005074A		
B DOE JANE S	02	222004433		1135
C				

63 TREATMENT AUTHORIZATION CODES	64 DOCUMENT CONTROL NUMBER	65 EMPLOYER NAME
A		
B		
C		

66 DX 3669	4019	79431												68

69 ADMIT DX 3669	70 PATIENT REASON DX a b c	71 PPS CODE	72 ECI a b c	73

74 PRINCIPAL PROCEDURE CODE DATE	a. OTHER PROCEDURE CODE DATE	b. OTHER PROCEDURE CODE DATE	75	76 ATTENDING NPI 29993745453	QUAL
153 09112007				LAST JONES FIRST JOHN J	
c. OTHER PROCEDURE CODE DATE	d. OTHER PROCEDURE CODE DATE	e. OTHER PROCEDURE CODE DATE		77 OPERATING NPI	QUAL
				LAST FIRST	

80 REMARKS	81CC a	78 OTHER NPI	QUAL
	b	LAST FIRST	
	c	79 OTHER NPI	QUAL
	d	LAST FIRST	

UB-04 CMS-1450   APPROVED OMB NO. 0938-0997   NUBC National Uniform Billing Committee   THE CERTIFICATIONS ON THE REVERSE APPLY TO THIS BILL AND ARE MADE A PART HEREOF.

FIGURE 3-1 UB-04 with information entered for John T. Doe, an outpatient of Jones Hospital

EDI#: 00120
Billing Provider: Jones Hospital
Medicare Provider #330127
Address: Barkley Building 225 Main Street Centerville, PA 17111
Attending Physician: John J Jones
NPI# 2999374543
Patient Account Number: 756048Q
Date of Admission: 09/11/2007
Statement Period Date: 09/11/2007 – 09/11/2007
Place of Service: Inpatient Hospital
Occurrence Codes and Dates:

A1 11/11/1936

A2 11/01/1991

B1 11/11/1936

B2 01/01/1987

Condition codes: 09
Value Codes: A2 $15.31
ICD-9 Procedure Codes and Dates: 15.3, 09/11/2007
Principal Diagnosis Code: 366.9
Secondary Diagnosis Codes: 401.9, 794.31
Number of Covered Days: 1
Services: Institutional Services Rendered:
Revenue Code: 305 HCPCS Procedure Code: 85025 Unit 1 Price $13.39
Revenue Code: 730 HCPCS Procedure Code: 93005 Unit 1 Price $76.54
Total Charges $89.93
Secondary Payer Subscriber: Jane S Doe (wife)
Subscriber Address: 125 City Avenue Centerville PA 17111
Sex: M
DOB: 11/11/1936
State Teachers ID# 222004433
Payer ID #: 1135

Here is the complete Data String with each separate line as the computer writes it.

```
ST*837*987654~
BHT*0019*00*0123*20070918*0932*CH~
REF*87*004010X96~
NM1*40*2*MEDICARE*****46*00120~
PER*IC*JANE DOE*TE*9005555555~
NM1*41*2*JONES HOSPITAL*****46*12345~
HL*1**20*1~
```

```
PRV*BI*ZZ*203BA0200N~
NM1*85*2*JONES HOSPITAL*****XX*330127~
PRV*AT*ZZ*363LP0200N~
N3*BARKLEY BUILDING 225 MAIN STREET~
N4*CENTERVILLE*PA*17111~
REF*G2*987654080~
HL*2*1*22*0~
SBR*P*18*******MB~
NM1*IL*1*DOE*JOHN*T***MI*030005074A~
N3*125 CITY AVENUE~
N4*CENTERVILLE*PA*17111~
DMG*D8*19361111*M~
NM1*PR*2*MEDICARE B*****PI*00435~
CLM*756048Q*89.93***14:A:1**Y*Y*Y~
DTP*434*D8*20070911~
CL1*3*1~
HI*BK:366.9~
HI*BF:401.9*BF:794.31~
HI*BQ:15.3:D8:20070911~
HI*BH:A1:D8:19361111*BH:A2:D8:19911101*BH:B1:D8:19361111*BH:B2:D8:19870101~
HI*BE:A2:::15.31~
HI*BG:09~
NM1*71*1*JONES*JOHN*J***XX*2999374543~
PRV*AT*ZZ*363LP0200N~
SBR*S*01*351630*STATE TEACHERS*GP****CI~
DMG***F~
OI***Y***Y~
NM1*IL*1*DOE*JANE*S***MI*222004433~
N3*125 CITY AVENUE~
N4*CENTERVILLE*PA*17111~
NM1*PR*2*STATE TEACHERS*****PI*1135~
LX*1~
SV2*305*HC:85025*13.39*UN*1~
DTP*472*D8*20070911~
LX*2~
SV2*730*HC:93005*76.54*UN*3~
DTP*472*D8*20070911~
SE*44*987654~
```

Each line begins with a computer code identifying the type of instruction. The end of each line finishes with a tilde (~). Looking through these lines of data, the billing specialist can find the Medicare ID number and the name and address of the service facility, among other information familiar to an insurance claim. Also listed are diagnosis codes, procedures, and their charges. Listed is the secondary insurance under Jane S. Doe with State Teachers insurance. The "header" lines are the first three beginning with "ST," "BHT," and "REF." These instructions begin the transaction and define the hierarchical type and the transmission type. At the end, or the caboose, is the "trailer" instruction beginning with "SE." This instructs the computer that the transaction is over and to prepare to begin the next claim.

The next example is the data string as the computer records it. The data string is one long line transmitted without any spaces or line breaks. Once the billing specialist knows the ending markings and separators, he or she can begin to understand the information and correct errors when they occur. At the provider office, the data string is not usually printed. This sample gives the reader an idea of just what is sent electronically and what the EDI data stream looks like.

```
ST*837*987654~BHT*0019*00*0123*20070918*0932*CH~REF*87*004010 X96~NM1*40*2*
MEDICARE*****46*00120~PER*IC*JANEDOE*TE*9005555555~NM1*41*2*JONESHOSPITAL*
****46*12345~HL*1**20*1~PRV*BI*ZZ*203BA0200N~NM1*85*2*JONES HOSPITAL*****
XX*330127~PRV*AT*ZZ*363LP0200N~N3*BARKLEYBUILDING 225 MAIN STREET~N4*CENTER
VILLE*PA*17111~REF*G2*987654080~HL*2*1*22*0~SBR*P*18******MB~NM1*IL*1*DOE
*JOHN*T***MI*030005074A~N3*125 CITY AVENUE~N4*CENTERVILLE*PA*17111~DMG*D8*
19361111*M~NM1*PR*2*MEDICARE B*****PI*00435~CLM*756048Q*89.93***14:A:1**Y*Y
*Y~DTP*434*D8*20070911~CL1*3*1~HI*BK:366.9~HI*BF:401.9*BF:794.31~HI*BQ:15.3:
D8:20070911~HI*BH:A1:D8:19361111*BH:A2:D8:19911101*BH:B1:D8:19361111*BH:B2
:D8:19870101~HI*BE:A2:::15.31~HI*BG:09~NM1*71*1*JONES*JOHN*J***XX*2999374
543~PRV*AT*ZZ*363LP0200N~SBR*S*01*351630*STATETEACHERS*GP****CI~DMG***F~OI
***Y***Y~NM1*IL*1*DOE*JANE*S***MI*222004433~N3*125 CITYAVENUE~N4*CENTERVIL
LE*PA*17111~NM1*PR*2*STATETEACHERS*****PI*1135~LX*1~SV2*305*HC:85025*13.39
*UN*1~DTP*472*D8*20070911~LX*2~SV2*730*HC:93005* 76.54*UN*3~DTP*472*D8*20
070911~SE*44*987654~
```

THINK ABOUT IT

This data stream is just too hard to figure out. As billing specialist, don't software programs translate this data stream into the claim formats?

LIMITATIONS OF ELECTRONIC CLAIMS

Most insurance claims can be submitted electronically. However, there are still occasions where a paper attachment is necessary to fully explain the reasons for the charges listed. At this writing, the DHHS has not completed the adoption of a standard for attachments to claims transactions. The organization Health Level Seven (HL7) is responsible to develop this standard. Until those standards are fully implemented, claims that require full attachments will still be accepted on paper.

A limitation to an electronic health claim is the size of the file, or loop iterations. The Transaction and Code Sets Rule stipulates the limit of 99 service lines in a professional claim. This is quite sufficient for most claims. A health plan must be able to accept that number of lines when presented to them electronically. They cannot delay or deny processing a claim as long as it complies with the HIPAA Transaction and Code Sets Rule.

REMITTANCE ADVICE AND SECONDARY PAYER

The original Health Care Claim X12N 837 form is used to send information to each health plan that covers the patient and lists the services rendered. The Health Care Claim Payment/Advice ASC X12N 835 returns information to the health care provider regarding payment and adjustment of payment. Some insurance claims are **crossover claims**, going to more than one health plan. Each health plan and insured has their own set of benefits. Under HIPAA, each plan must accept and process any transaction that meets the national standard. Each health plan listing the patient as a beneficiary will receive the same information and must process the claim in a timely manner. This allows for coordination of benefits with each responsible health plan. The transmission of the claim will not be returned to the provider until each health plan has had a chance to respond with their remittance advice. The health care provider is not to be penalized or the claim delayed when the payer receives claims for services they do not cover.

All claims must be processed, no matter the content of the claim. Perhaps the charges included are not part of the coverage they offer this particular patient. But the secondary payer, or possibly third payer, does cover these charges. For example, prior to HIPAA, Medicare would accept claims for their covered services and reject all others. Now Medicare must forego that policy and process all claims that meet HIPAA specifications. This does not mean that Medicare, or any other health plan, has to change their payment policy. Medicare does not pay for a face-lift for cosmetic purposes only. With HIPAA standards implemented, Medicare is required to accept and process the bill, but still will not pay for a face-lift that is purely for cosmetic purposes. (FAQs, 2003). Medicare will pass the claim electronically to the next payer for their review. Perhaps their benefits include payment at least in part for a face-lift for cosmetic purposes. The secondary or other payer will be able to make their determination about their reimbursement from the electronic information provided.

Prior to the Transaction and Code Sets Rule, a provider would send a claim with the information that only pertained to that first payer. After receiving the remittance advice, the provider would adjust the claim to meet the specific information needs for the secondary payer, add a photo-copy of the remittance advice, then mail the newly adjusted claim to the second payer. This procedure was repeated if a third payer was listed. Under HIPAA, the health care provider is to include all information for all payers needed to adjudicate the health plan's claim. As stated in HIPAA law, each health plan receiving a standard transmission is not to delete any information given them even though it is not important for the adjudication of their claim. That is administrative simplification in action.

Let's look at another example. One plan pays for a portion of home health services while another may not include that benefit. In compliance with HIPAA, they must accept the transmission with all the home health data. The payer cannot up-front reject such a claim. The payer is not required to bring that data into their adjudication system and provide payment. The payer, acting in accordance with policy and contractual agreements, can ignore data within the X12N 837 data set and pass the information on to the secondary payer.

Working with Outside Entities

All health care providers need to have close communication with health plans that they transact business with electronically. The health plan and the health care provider are referred to as **trading partners**. Various types of trading partners are hospitals; physicians; health care payers such as insurance companies; health maintenance organizations (HMOs); pre-ferred provider organizations (PPOs); local, state, and federal govern-mental authorities; and trade organizations such as hospital associations. These entities may also be business associates of each other. Health care providers may have a written trading partner agreement with each of their trading partners. This is *not* a requirement of HIPAA law. It functions as protection between the health plan and health care provider so both parties understand the terms of partnership. In HIPAA, this concept only details the use of electronic transactions and code set standards. The rule does not explain how the transaction is to be sent or received or what is done with the transaction after receipt. This is where an agreement will specify EDI processing functions and requirements. If covered entities enter into a trading partner agreement (TPA), HIPAA law outlines certain restrictions placed on such agreements.

Trading Partner Agreements

The agreement to conduct business electronically in order to transmit e-PHI is called a **trading partner agreement (TPA)**. The written document is an agreement related to the exchange of information in electronic transactions between each party. This definition allows for other arrangements to be formed between the two parties. TPAs may not modify or add or change the meaning of any values transmitted other than what is defined by the HIPAA Standards for Electronic Transactions. Both parties agree not to change any data element or segment to suit particular situations, nor change the order in which segments are delivered between themselves. TPA also must agree *not* to utilize any code or data in a manner that is unique to their communication. The HIPAA officer is responsible for defining these agreements. The HIPAA officer must remember that if someone else is depended on for technical advice, the officer must make sure that the vendor is doing reliable work. It is the health care provider's security officer who is responsible to the CMS concerning compliance, not the software vendor. Payers are required by law to have the capability to send and receive all HIPAA transactions. Thus, it encourages trading partners to be clear about the specific data within the 837 transmissions they require or would prefer to have in order to efficiently adjudicate their claim. (ASC X12N Guide, 2000). Typical TPAs would cover subjects such as provider identifiers, processing requirements, provider taxonomy codes, situational issues, and intercommunications, testing, and contact information.

Business Use and Definition

The ASC X12N standards minimize the need for users to reprogram their data processing systems for multiple formats. This is a driving force behind the Administrative Simplification portion of HIPAA. The transmission standards *do not* define the method in which the interchange with trading partners is to take place. The link between hardware and translation software is flexible within the stated guidelines. The ASC success with other business and industry applications validates the simplicity of the open architecture format with wide variations in application. Each trading partner, which will interface with another trading partner, must meet HIPAA requirements individually.

ENFORCEMENT OF TRANSACTIONS AND CODE SETS

Change in any form can be difficult. HIPAA mandated that all health plans receive claims in the exact same format as every other health plan. This limited some of the information they received that had become part of their adjudication process. Prior to HIPAA, many health plans required supplemental information on separate forms in order to process claims. Other health plans insisted that providers follow specific instructions in certain blocks on the claim form. This meant that claims had to be revised when there was more than one payer. Insurance companies began to seek ways to insert some of that missing information into the standard transaction. In a standard transaction, there are "optional" data fields. Payers appropriated some of these and required providers to supply certain information they felt important to process their claim. As early as two years after implementation, the Workgroup for Electronic Data Interchange (WEDI) found a number of these additional fields being used—even among some government plans. The payers explained the requirements in "companion guides" to the transaction guides. WPC is the approved publisher of standard transaction implementation guides. Health care providers were soon forced to obtain "companion implementation guides" for each specific health plan that insisted on changing the transaction format. These types of adjustments thwart the interoperability of standard transactions. It makes the coordination of benefits between plans all but impossible. (Bazzoli, 2004). This "adjustment" is also in violation of the Transaction and Code Sets Rule. It is contrary to the trading partner agreements that should be in place.

If a health care provider finds a health plan, for example, wanting to adjust a data element to suit their needs, the security officer may submit a HIPAA Non-Privacy Complaint. Complaint forms are accessible from the CMS Web site for downloading and printing. The **Office of E-Health Standards and Services (OESS)** is the branch of CMS overseeing these complaints. The complaint may be sent via mail or electronically. The electronic version is found at the CMS Web site, http://cms/hhs.gov. Search for HIPAA complaint, Non-Privacy Complaint Form. If the complaint relates to a transaction or code sets, list the transaction involved and the type of complaint as follows:

1. Noncompliant transaction received

2. Compliant transaction sent and rejected

3. Code set received or sent and rejected

Other alleged violations relate to the disclosure of e-PHI. This form covers these as well. Appendix C has a copy of the printable form of HIPAA Non-Privacy Complaint Form.

The DHHS has set up the **Office of HIPAA Standards (OHS),** within the CMS, specifically to address the enforcement of the HIPAA Transactions and Code Sets Rule. This office operates independently from CMS to oversee compliance. (What is the HIPAA Office of HIPAA Standards?, 2004). As with the Privacy Rule, the CMS will look for voluntary compliance and expect to find good faith effort to comply with the standards. If failure to comply is based on reasonable cause and is not due to willful neglect, the HHS may not impose a civil monetary penalty. The department would expect the organization to submit compliance plans and show improvement after a 30-day period. Fines and penalties are part of the Correction Action Plan outlined by the secretary of DHHS. If the OHS finds possible criminal violations, they will direct the Department of Justice to investigate. (Guidance on Compliance with HIPAA Transaction and Code Sets, 2003).

SUMMARY

The HIPAA legislation mandates that when a health care provider and health plan communicate e-PHI electronically, the transmission must comply with certain ASC X12N standards. In order to be sure that any health care provider has the resources to send claims to any health plan, a uniform standard transaction is used. The DHHS looked to industry standards endorsed by the Accredited Standards Committee. The DHHS took the X12N transmissions designed by and for the insurance industry and added some file standards to fit the purposes of transmitting e-PHI. There are eight standard transactions that are endorsed by the DHHS that are to be used by health plans and health care providers as well as health care clearinghouses.

In order to standardize transactions, all parties must use the same *language,* or code sets, to communicate with each other. The medical code sets adopted are those generally in use prior to HIPAA law. The ICD-9-CM Vols.1 and 2 are adopted to code diagnoses. The Volume 3 of ICD-9-CM is designated to code inpatient procedures. Two standards are adopted to code physician and nonphysician procedures for outpatients: CPT-4 and HCPCS Level II. Dental procedures are to be coded from the CDT-4 book. Drugs are coded from the National Drug Code System. Each of these is updated regularly, and only current codes are to be used. Nonmedical codes needed to communicate with other information in code form were adopted. These originate with the DHHS.

The eight transactions include claim forms; payment and remittance advice; inquiry and responses for eligibility; inquiry and response for determining the status of a particular claim; request for review to determine coverage and extent of reimbursement; and inquiry concerning enrollment status of a patient. The data sent electronically is in computer format yet is human readable. Errors in data can be found since the sequence of information is uniform and separators help locate invalid entries. Since all health plans can receive claims electronically, this allows for crossover claims to be transmitted electronically. Coordination of benefits is easy since all information is included in the first claim transmission. There is a transaction form under development by the Health Level 7 organization for claims attachments.

Each health care provider and health plan has the option of trading partner agreements, though this is not mandated by HIPAA. Trading partners are to abide by HIPAA law and not change any portion of electronic transmissions to suit their particular needs. The Office of HIPAA Standards under the CMS is the designated enforcement agency for the DHHS. The OHS will look to the health care provider for compliance, not the software vendor. Each HIPAA officer needs to be sure his or her office software is compliant since the responsibility rests with him or her.

REVIEW QUESTIONS

1. How does the Transaction and Code Sets portion of HIPAA demonstrate real administrative simplification?

2. What added responsibilities does the Transaction and Code Sets Rule place on the HIPAA security officer? Which segments of the health care staff are involved with the Transaction and Code Sets Rule?

3. Prior to HIPAA, each health plan had the opportunity to request specific information to process a claim. Why was it necessary to eliminate the differences with the ASC X12 standards?

4. Transaction and Code Sets Rule mandates that no health plan can reject a claim in the X12N format. What restriction is placed on the health plan about any information included in the standard transaction that is not important to its adjudication?

5. When a state Medicaid plan enters into a contract with a managed care organization (MCO) to provide services to Medicaid recipients, that organization in turn contracts with specific health care providers to render the services. When a health care provider submits encounter information electronically to the managed care organization, is this activity required to be a standard transaction?

6. Assume, the managed care organization (MCO) then submits a bill to the state Medicaid agency for payment for all the care given to all the persons covered by that managed care organization (MCO) for that month under a capitation agreement. Should this be a standard transaction?

7. List advantages of having crossover claims with complete information for each health plan sent in one transmission rather than returning each time to the provider.

8. Decide whether each of these is an example of a trading partner (TP), a business associate (BA), or both trading partner and business associate (TPBA).

   a) _____A health care provider and a software vendor

   b) _____A health care provider and a health insurance company

   c) _____A health care provider and a pharmacy

   d) _____A health care provider and an outside laboratory

   e) _____A health care provider and a cleaning service for the office

9. If our office finds that a trading partner wants to change one of the data elements to include information pertaining to their system, what should our office do?

10. Discuss why full disclosure of physician notes or reports is contrary to the "minimum necessary" concept of the Privacy Rule.

11. The claims attachment transaction X12 N 275, which is under development, asks for specific information rather than complete reports. This has reduced the need for written attachments in its pilot run. There is concern in the industry about this format. The health care industry is divided on this. What are some pros and cons of this issue?

References

Administrative Simplification Compliance Act (ASCA) Enforcement of Mandatory Electronic Submission of Medicare Claims, Medicare Learning Network Matters Number: MM3440 (January 27, 2005). Retrieved April 26, 2007, from http://www.cms.hhs.gov/MLNMattersArticles/downloads/MM3440.pdf.

American Psychiatric Association. (2004, October 1). *DSM-IV-TR October 1 coding alert*. Retrieved July 15, 2006, from http://www.dsm4tr.org/coding/cfm.

ASC X12N insurance subcommittee implementation guide. (May 2000). Pp. A1 and 13.

Bazzoli, Fred. (2004, March). WEDI warns of "glaring" HIPAA errors. *Healthcare IT NewsWeek*, p. 1.

Final Regulation Text: Standards for Electronic Transactions. (2000, July 25, last modified Friday, January 31, 2003). Retrieved May 17, 2003, from http://www.cms.hhs.gov/hipaa/hipaa2/regulations/transactions/ finalrule/txfin01.asp.

Frequently Asked Questions about Electronic Transactions Standards Adopted under HIPAA, (September 8, 2003, updated September 8, 2000). Retrieved from http://www.aspe.hhs.gov/admnsimp/faqtx.htm, p. 6.

Guidance on Compliance with HIPAA Transaction and Code Sets. (July 23, 2003). Retrieved from http://www.cms.gov.

Health Insurance Reform: Modifications to Electronic Data Transaction Standards and Code Sets, Final Rule. 68 Fed.Reg. 8,381–8,399 (February 20, 2003) (to codify 45 C.F.R. pt. 162).

Health Insurance Reform: Standards for Electronic Transactions, Final Rule. 65 Fed.Reg. 50,312–50,372 (August 17, 2000) (to codify 45 C.F.R. pts. 160, 162).

HIPAA Administrative Simplification: Standards for Electronic Health Care Claims Attachments, Proposed Rule, 70 Fed. Reg. 55,990–55,999 (September 23, 2005).

What is the Office of HIPAA Standards? Answer ID 2610, HIPAA Administrative Simplification (January 23, 2004). Retrieved from http://questions.cms.hhs.gov/cgi-bin/cmshhs.cfg/php.

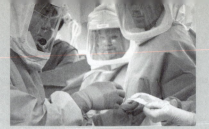

CHAPTER

4

SECURITY RULE EXPLAINED

OBJECTIVES

Describe the need for safeguards of electronic protected health information (e-PHI).

Understand the basics of administrative safeguards, physical safeguards, and technical safeguards for e-PHI.

Identify the role of the HIPAA security officer as responsible for local training and enforcing of HIPAA regulations.

Explain the government's role in overseeing compliance and setting up means to file a complaint.

KEY TERMS

---

access

administrative safeguards

algorithm

audit trail

authentication

contingency plan

electronic protected health information, (e-PHI)

encryption

information system

infrastructure

integrity

nonrepudiation

password

physical safeguards

risk

risk analysis

risk management

security of electronic protected health information

security incident

technical safeguards

user

workstation

INTRODUCTION

*The Security Rule addresses the issue of keeping **electronic protected health information (e-PHI)** from unauthorized disclosures as well as guarding against possible threats and loss. This rule considers security to be different from privacy. To ensure electronic privacy, there must be high levels of security measures in place so unauthorized individuals do not gain access to information that is considered private. **Access** is considered the exposure necessary to read, write, modify, or communicate data and information. Access privilege is what allows an individual to enter a computer system for an authorized purpose. To provide and maintain the **security of electronic protected health information** (e-PHI) means there are safeguards in an information system that protect it, its data, and information against unauthorized access and limit access to authorized users in accordance with an established policy. Security also means protecting the **integrity** of the data system, i.e., protecting the data against unauthorized alteration. Each covered entity must have hardware and software equipment in place that maintains integrity of the data as well as protects against loss, i.e., backups. Safeguards cost money and time to install and then to administer. The government has mandated five topics that each covered entity is to address in order to provide security for the e-PHI they handle. These topics are 1) administrative safeguards, 2) physical safeguards, 3) technical safeguards, 4) organization requirement, and lastly, 5) policies, procedures, and documentation. Some of these concepts change the way business is conducted in the health care workplace. It is important that each staff member be aware of the measures needed to keep their data secure. The Security Rule relies heavily on good technical support and expertise to keep the flow of information moving securely.*

THINK ABOUT IT

1. Do privacy and security mean the same thing?
2. If a person's PHI is kept private, isn't it also secure?

CORE REQUIREMENTS

The Department of Health and Human Services (DHHS) has moved into the next phase of "accountability" in regard to e-PHI—that of ensuring the security of the e-PHI that a covered entity maintains. Prior to HIPAA, paper copies of medical records were handled in a restricted manner to protect each patient's privacy. But little was done to provide backup copies in case of loss, disaster recovery, or off-site storage. Certainly privacy and security are closely related. Protecting the privacy of electronic information depends largely on the existence of security measures, yet security covers much more. The Privacy Rule sets standards for disclosure and usage of paper-based PHI. It restricts when, how, and how much health information can be provided when authorized. The new issue of security comes with the move to electronic health information. There are many stories of computer hackers who access databases containing personal information of all kinds. The health care industry is particularly concerned about securing individually identifiable health information (IIHI). Information about mental health status, HIV/AIDS condition, or any other health status of an individual could end up in someone's possession without authorization if appropriate care is not taken. A disgruntled employee can misuse health information to discredit a coworker. An estranged marriage partner, jealous or greedy family members, or business associates are other examples of individuals who can use protected health information dishonestly. By standardizing the requirement to secure health information, the DHHS believes every individual will be able to know that his or her personal health information is private *and* secure. There is a difference between keeping e-PHI private and keeping e-PHI secure. *All* PHI, no matter whether electronic, oral, paper, film, report, etc., must be protected and kept *private*. All PHI in *electronic* form, e-PHI, must also be kept *secure*. The focus of the Security Rule is on electronic information and ways it is protected from alteration, accidental disclosure, or loss.

Health information can be in many forms that use electronic hardware. Methods of transferring information such as paper-to-paper faxes, person-to-person telephone calls, unrecorded video teleconferencing, and voice mail messages are *not* subject to the Security Rule—even though they may contain electronic memory and can produce multiple copies. This list of excluded items also includes fax-back and voice response systems. A "fax-back" system is when a request for information is made via voice using a fax machine. The requested information is returned as a fax-back. The HIPAA Security Ruling covers *electronic* medical record systems and *electronic* order entry systems. That is, the data is stored in databases, text files, digital pictures, or any other binary format systems using computer storage media. The Security Rule also covers all binary *transmissions* of data.

All health care providers must be sure they comply with the Security Ruling in four core areas.

1. *Confidentiality, integrity, and availability* of all electronic protected health information (e-PHI) they create, receive, maintain, or transmit

2. *Protecting against anticipated uses or disclosures* of electronic information that are not permitted or required under the Privacy Rule

3. *Protecting against any anticipated threats or hazards* to the security, survivability, and integrity of electronic protected health information (e-PHI)

4. *Ensuring compliance* with the Security Rule by their workforce. (Ernst & Young, 2003)

Requirements are organized into five categories: administrative, physical, technical safeguards, organizational requirements, and policies, procedures, and documentation. We will study each of these categories. In a lot of ways privacy and security are interrelated. When a covered entity works for compliance with the Privacy Ruling, they also comply with certain areas of the Security Ruling. But keeping e-PHI private does not necessarily mean it is fully secure. The DHHS covered many areas to be sure information is secure. Since this ruling applies to small one-physician offices and large multicampus teaching hospitals, the rules allow for a lot of interpretation to meet the situation. However, every entity *must* meet certain standards while other requirements in the final plan can be adjusted. In other words, some security issues are listed as required and some issues are "addressable." The required items must be achieved and documented. Addressable items must be considered and solutions documented that are "reasonable and appropriate" for the particular entity. Where a health care provider finds a security issue that for them is not "reasonable and appropriate," the covered entity must document that decision of noncompliance and explain why it is not reasonable or appropriate for them. Documentation must include what the health care provider will substitute as an alternative policy or procedure in order to achieve the same goal. In all cases the covered entity must *document* what they are doing or why they are not doing it if they choose not to comply. See Appendix D for a chart from the Centers for Medicare and Medicaid (CMS) Web site showing items that are required and those that are addressable.

Administrative Safeguards

The DHHS sets the standard but does not specify how to comply. The Security Rule mandates that each covered entity appoint someone to be responsible for securing e-PHI. It includes administrative actions plus policies and procedures to manage the selection, development, implementation, and maintenance of security measures to protect e-PHI. The administrative safeguards also include managing the conduct of the covered entity's workforce in relation to the protection of that information. During an audit, the Centers for Medicare and Medicaid Services (CMS) will ask to see procedures and policies that outline how the entity is meeting the administrative safeguard requirements of the Security Rule. These areas are the following:

- Security management
- Assigned security responsibility
- Workforce security
- Information access
- Security awareness and training
- Security incidents
- Contingency plans
- Evaluation of security effectiveness
- Business associate contracts

Security Management

The process of *security management* involves implementing policies and procedures to prevent, detect, and contain any intrusions of security. This is a required part of the Security Rule. The HIPAA officer or designated security officer (further explanation of this position to follow) is to conduct and maintain a risk analysis of the provider's organization. Before a health care provider can understand what they need to do to comply with the Security Rule, they must find out where the threats are to e-PHI. The administrator considers the cost of various security and control measures against the losses that would be expected if these measures were not in place. Each health care provider must look at the areas where e-PHI could be disclosed, altered, or lost in a way that is contrary to the Security Rule. The investigation must follow the path of electronic data and test each type of storage or movement of data for any problems. The concept of **risk** is quite broad. It includes the impact and likelihood of an adverse event—the possibility of harm or loss to any software, information, hardware, administrative, physical, communications, or personnel resource within an automated information system or activity. That makes the administrator's responsibility to conduct a risk analysis quite a task. The **risk analysis** focuses on the security of the computer system and the identification of critical data (criticality). The security officer must consider what cost-effective security and control measures may be selected to balance the cost of these security control measures against the losses that would be expected if these measures were not in place. Once the risk analysis is completed, the covered entity must write a plan to manage and minimize the risks they encountered. **Risk management** is the ongoing process that calculates the risk of loss or disclosure of electronic information. Security measures are managed to offset threats and the vulnerability of e-PHI to a minimal, acceptable amount.

The risk analysis asks some important questions like these:

- Who is able to view what information?

- Are there limits to the amount of information accessed by employees?

- Is it kept to the "minimum necessary"?

- Is there opportunity for the public or patients to view e-PHI other than their own?

- How could this data be lost?

- What is the impact if the data cannot be recovered?

- What if it were sent to the wrong party?

- How could it be altered in an unauthorized manner?

This investigation forms the basis for determining what areas need to be adjusted within the covered entity. The risk analysis must be written to comply with the rule. The study to find problems or gaps between current practices and what the Security Rule requires is called a *gap analysis*. Each health care provider must look at the measures they already have in place to provide security and reduce risks, then compare that to the additional measures they need to take to reach the level of compliance the Security Rule requires—the gap between current status and compliance with Security Rule. An *adverse threat* is a transmission of e-PHI that is not secure with the result that information could be stolen, lost, or received by some party other than the intended entity. Any risks that are found must be documented. Once the risks are found, the next step is to decide how to manage those risks or to put hardware, software, and policies in place to minimize the risk to near zero. The goal is to bring risks of disclosure or loss to a reasonable and bare minimum level. If the CMS requests a review of policy, the agents will expect to find a documented risk analysis as the first item completed for compliance. The management portion of the security protections is meant to be scalable and flexible, so whether small or large, the covered entity can find a way to comply with the ruling. Cost considerations to bring the organization into compliance are also to be part of the decision making process. These rulings are not funded—the government has not allowed for covered entities to receive payment for the mandated changes. Since each entity is to work toward compliance, the covered entity is expected to move in that direction and find a way they can pay for the changes.

Assigned Security Responsibility—Security Officer

The administrator of each health care entity is to appoint a *security officer* whose responsibility is to develop and implement the policies and procedures required by the HIPAA Security Rule. This may be the same person as the privacy officer or the HIPAA officer mentioned in earlier chapters. The CMS looks to the security officer as the one responsible within the organization to administer and manage security compliance. The officer is to take the *gap analysis*—the difference between where the entity stands on compliance and where they need to be according to the Security Rule—and make recommendations for change and see to it that changes are made. The workforce must be trained in ways that ensure security measures are followed and limits to access are in place. The security officer is the one to oversee the management and supervision of persons in the workforce in relation to e-PHI security issues. The security officer or designated person is to regularly review audit logs and other security tracking reports. Logs are used to record who accessed electronic health information and when it was accessed. The security officer will need to periodically check for security threats or gaps as new equipment is brought in or software programs are updated. Another area for the security officer to check is the Human Resource Department as employees leave the workforce or move from one department to another. Passwords and access to certain information need to be adjusted as employees change responsibilities. This standard is required.

Workforce Security

The responsibility of continued security within the workforce includes maintaining a record of access authorizations. The security officer must ensure that personnel operating and maintaining data systems have proper access authorization. When finished doing maintenance work, the maintenance access must be closed. Establishing personnel clearance procedures, establishing and maintaining security policies and procedures, and ensuring that system users have proper training are appropriate activities toward meeting the requirements. A **user** is a person with authorized access to the computer system. **Passwords** are a confidential alphanumeric string used in conjunction with a user name to verify the identity of the individual attempting to gain access to a computer system. Other things such as changing combination locks, removing a name from access lists, removing user account(s), and turning in keys, tokens, or swipe cards that allow access are necessary to maintain the integrity of the security system as employees leave or move to a different department. The integrity of the system must be maintained to ensure data or information has not been altered or destroyed in an unauthorized manner. It is necessary to change the authorization and delete or change passwords to prevent unauthorized access to electronic information. A regular schedule of new passwords aids in keeping the system secure. Staff should be trained to resist "social engineering," a form of phishing for private data, such as access codes. For example, a person who appears to be legitimate might approach a vulnerable staff member asking for a password to "test something." A recent rash of phony Joint Commission surveyors has raised the issue to a new threat level.

This standard is addressable. Each entity determines what fits. Some providers have implemented biotechnology for security. A small provider may find this too expensive. There is no one solution to address these items. The security procedures are to be documented, and in that manner, the entity is considered in compliance.

Information Access

Each covered entity must have policies in place for implementing and maintaining the appropriate level of access for all personnel authorized to view health information. This standard is required. Each job description carries with it an explanation of the extent of information needed to perform that job adequately. Access should be limited to the minimum necessary, as with the Privacy Rule. The access should not restrict anyone from completing his or her job responsibilities relating to health care, billing, or normal operations.

The following true story is an example of someone with authorized access to e-PHI telling someone within the facility information that might have seemed good for the protection of others. However, disclosure of information in relation to conditions like AIDS is specifically protected and must have proper authorization from the patient.

TRUE STORY

A physician was diagnosed with AIDS at the hospital in which he practiced medicine. His surgical privileges were suspended. (Estate of Behringer v. Medical Center at Princeton, 1991).

1.   *Why is this a security issue, not just a privacy issue?*
2.   *Do credentialing personnel, who might know this type of information, violate the staff member's privacy? Was security weak?*

Security Awareness and Training

Training is important for all workforce employees and nonemployees like physicians and volunteers. Training should include administration personnel, too, since they have access to electronic information. The training is to stimulate awareness about the vulnerability of data within the electronic system and ways to ensure its safety. The workforce ought to know about virus protection measures. Training should include how to immediately report any event that might mean the protection has been compromised. Proper login and logoff procedure lessens the possibility of unauthorized access to health information. Training should include password usage and proper changes of passwords to ensure the safety of the system. Sharing passwords is by far the most common security violation. Training is to be done periodically. The Security Rule says that security training is required for all staff and is to be reasonable and appropriate to carrying out their functions in the facility. Periodic retraining should be given whenever environmental or operational changes affect the security of e-PHI. The rule requires the security officer to retain records of this training for six years. Six years coincides with the time frame for civil monetary penalties. (Health Insurance Reform, 2003)

Since each health care provider is different, this standard is addressable. Each security officer is to meet the standard for training and awareness as it best fits his or her organization.

Security Incidents

A **security incident** is defined as the attempted or successful unauthorized access, use, disclosure, modification, destruction of information, or interference with system operations in an **information system**. An information system normally includes hardware, software, information, data, applications, communications, and people. Yes, data is different from information. Data consists of elements that when rearranged or summarized into a report become information. It interconnects information resources under the same direct management control that shares a common functionality or purpose. The DHHS defines this attempted or successful unauthorized access into an information system a security incident rather than a security breach. Protected health information may not have been compromised but the possibility exists—hence, the word *incident*. This is a required standard. The story above is just one of many recorded examples of how manipulation of software access allowed e-PHI to be open to Internet access. This incident was not intentional, but the implications of this incident could be very damaging to specific individuals.

In response to an incident, HIPAA Security Rule mandates that there be a formal, documented response executed and a report written. The security incident must be included in the medical records of each affected individual. Besides that, all patients must be notified in writing of the incident. Notification of patients protects the covered entity from accusations of hiding the access. It allows each patient to know of the incident so they are aware if someone uses information against them. All covered entity workers are expected to report a security incident no matter what the size or origin. The health care provider is better off taking steps early to protect information and prevent a larger problem. This minimizes exposure and will help e-PHI from being broadcast further. Sometimes the incident will involve another covered entity. Advising a covered entity immediately is part of expected business practice. This will help the other entity to contain the possible breach of security at their end and advise them of the need to report the incident too.

Contingency Plans

Many people ignore disaster plans and continuity planning. Perhaps a better term is business continuity. They perceive these to be very costly and difficult to manage. **Contingency planning**, now called *business continuity planning* for security, is defined as having policies and procedures in place to respond to an emergency or other occurrence that damages systems containing e-PHI. The reality of a disaster, whether very local or more widespread, is a possibility that needs planning for. No place has assurance against natural disasters. No one can guarantee against human-caused disaster either, and no one can protect completely against a terrorist attack. If disaster strikes, can individuals get access to their health information? Can information be accessed from an off-site location? Each covered entity must have a plan in place and maintain that plan as equipment and staff change.

Since there is no guarantee regarding disastrous emergencies, it is required that a contingency plan, or business continuity plan, be in place. Items in this plan include:

- Critical data analysis, i.e., what data is critical to operations?
- A data backup plan
- A disaster recovery plan
- An emergency mode operation plan
- Testing and revision procedures

Covered entities must consider how natural disasters could damage systems that contain e-PHI and develop policies and procedures for responding to such situations. Having backup data stored off-site and recycled on a regular basis is part of a contingency plan. Consideration should be given to how business can continue if it is not possible to continue work in the facility. What measures need to be taken to begin again in a new location, even temporarily?

Evaluation of Security Effectiveness

The HIPAA Security Rule requires that each covered entity periodically conduct an evaluation of their security safeguards. This periodic check will document its compliance with HIPAA on a routine basis. Any time there is new equipment brought on line, new software installed, or even an update of software, it should be evaluated as to its effectiveness and compliance with HIPAA. In this way, documentation of compliance will be current, and ready when needed.

Business Associate Contracts

Part of the business associate (BA) contract written under the Privacy Rule involves satisfactory assurance that the BA will appropriately safeguard e-PHI it receives and transmits. The security officer must review these contracts with BAs. All covered entities have worked out agreements to deal with the Privacy Rule. An appendix (addition) may be necessary to add wording to cover the Security Rule regulations. The contract between the covered entity and the business associate must provide that the business associate will:

- Implement safeguards that are reasonable and appropriate to protect the confidentiality, integrity, and availability of electronic protected health information it creates, receives, maintains, or transmits.

- Ensure that any agent (staff member) who may be entrusted with such information agrees to the same safeguards.

- Report to the covered entity *any* security incident of which it becomes aware.

- Authorize termination of the contract if the covered entity determines that the business associate has violated the contract.

Physical Safeguards

The next focus of security deals with equipment and the physical storage and maintenance of e-PHI. The **physical safeguards** include physical access measures, policies, and procedures to protect a covered entity's electronic information systems and related buildings and equipment from natural and environmental hazards and unauthorized intrusion. The items required under physical safeguards for security cover four areas.

1. Facility access controls: building, computers, and infrastructure closets

2. Workstation location and access

3. Workstation (software) security

4. Device and media controls

Facility Access Controls

Facility access deals with gaining entry to areas where e-PHI is stored and access to the physical location where computer hardware is located. The security officer must document how his or her particular organization is addressing physical access—the specifics are considered addressable. The specifics must include:

- Disaster recovery, business continuity

- Emergency mode operation

- A facility security plan

- Procedures for verifying access authorizations before any access is permitted

Access to computer information system hardware is to be limited to only those workers who need to administer and maintain the electronic systems where e-PHI is stored. Limiting access involves keeping doors locked and using keys or electronic locks. An advantage of electronic locks is their capability to log entries. Other items that need to be considered are the maintenance records, need-to-know procedures for personnel access, sign-in/sign-out record for visitors, and visitor escorts. A typical checklist to meet HIPAA Physical Security includes questions like these:

- How do you access the building?

- Are closed circuit cameras recording?

- Is there an employee entrance?

- Are the doors manual or electric?

- Can access be gained from the loading dock or garage?

- How do visitors gain access to the building?

- Are business visitors escorted at all times?

This last question considers business visitors different than patients and their guests. This refers to business visitors who may enter parts of the building where they would have access to equipment that holds and maintains e-PHI. This includes people coming for repair of equipment or facilities, salespeople, or inspectors. The Privacy Rule stipulates that a business agreement must be in force with these parties in case they access any e-PHI.

Some questions dealing with health information in the *patient care areas* are these:

- Are medical records stored securely?

- Are they protected from fire, loss, theft, etc.?

- Is e-PHI protected from incidental viewing by visitors?

The security officer must continuously provide reasonable safeguards for each of these situations and document them in the policy manual for security.

Workstation Use

The definition of **workstation** is an electronic computing device, for example, a laptop or desktop computer, a personal data assistant (PDA) or any other device that performs similar functions, and electronic media stored in its immediate environment. No matter where these are located inside or outside a facility, workstation access to information is to be limited to the job description. A workstation "log-off" procedure is very important to minimize unauthorized access to health information. Auto logoff is a requirement. Time delay is not specified, but a ten-minute delay to logoff is a good maximum and a *de facto* standard.

Workstation Security

Each person on the workforce should understand the Internet use policy as well as the e-mail policy of the entity. Equipment at the covered entity is to be used for business and not personal use. Personal use introduces a whole class of security risks. Training will include how to save computer files for best backup security and how to manage backup equipment. Some questions dealing with workstation security are these:

- Does the workforce understand how to lock their computer screen?

- Are passwords, tokens, or biometrics used to secure workstations?

- Can workstation screens be viewed by passers-by?

- Is any e-PHI stored on the workstation or user device?

Security standards extend to members of a provider's workforce, whether they work on site or at home. Any transcriptionists or other workers who have been authorized to work from their homes must have the same security protections as those employees working on site. "At home" workers are defined as part of a covered entity's workforce and are a special high risk. Information systems personnel must extend security to all off-site locations. Any security incidents must be reported and procedures followed to remedy the situation. These off-site locations must be protected and monitored just like on-site workstations.

Device and Media Controls

The security officer is to keep a record of the receipt and removal of all central processing unit (CPU) hardware and clinical software that is used within the facility. This provides a means to track when certain hardware items are purchased. When that item is considered obsolete or is not to be used any longer, the security officer must have a record of its disposition. Disks, tapes, handheld devices, text messaging and camera cell phones, video recorders, and similar electronic communication devices are also items that are covered by this portion of the ruling. Electronic devices can hold many pieces of e-PHI. The Security Rule requires that disposal and reuse of equipment and media be documented. This rule covers disposal of *all* forms of media that contain e-PHI. The information may be on backup tapes and disks and any memory equipment, as well as server disks. It can be on thermal transfer ribbons from fax machines and label printers. E-PHI is also on diagnostic images and CDs. The security officer needs to compile an inventory of all equipment containing e-PHI. Don't forget the digital camera used to document therapy or wounds. The list must have the date when it entered the system and when it was disposed of, how it was disposed of, and measures taken to delete any information that is protected. Just how the officer meets these standards is an addressable issue since each organization varies so much. These devices must be erased, deleted, or destroyed in an appropriate manner when discarded. This is to prevent them from being resold or recycled to members of the public who unknowingly receive information that should have been deleted, destroyed, or erased. This portion of the Security Rule addresses the problem illustrated by the following true story.

TRUE STORY

Confidential Medicaid records were disclosed during the sale of surplus equipment by the Arkansas Department of Human Services twice in six months. In October 2001, the state stopped the sale of the department's surplus computer storage drives when it was discovered that Medicaid records that were supposed to be erased were found on the computers. In April 2002, a man who bought a file cabinet from the department found the files of Medicaid clients in one of the cabinet's drawers. The files included four Social Security numbers and birth dates. (DHS Surplus Sales, 2002).

Technical Safeguards

Technical safeguards mean the technology and the policy and procedures for its use that protect e-PHI and control access to it. There are several areas relating to the **infrastructure** that need to be in place to ensure the security of e-PHI. The word "infrastructure" applies to the underlying foundation or basic framework of a system or organization. Here the infrastructure means the computer server(s), hubs, switches, connecting wires, terminals and desk units, and the rooms or closets where they are located that are part of the installation within the building. (Briggs, 2004). Many health care providers have extended infrastructures called WANs, or wide area networks. Access is also extended through virtual private networks, or VPNs. These must be kept secure from intrusion.

The security officer must address issues dealing with the following:

- Access control
- Audit controls
- Integrity (of electronic PHI)
- Person or entity authentication
- Transmission security

The DHHS includes a certification standard for technical systems and software that each covered entity must meet in order to be "compliant." The department does not define *how* to meet the requirements.

Access Control

Access control prevents unauthorized people (or unauthorized processes) from entering the information technology system. This is an addressable item for compliance. There are several methods to regulate access control: a personal identification number (PIN), a password system, or a biometric identification system. Biometric identification uses a part of the body to authenticate the individual such as iris of the eye, fingerprint shape recognition, or handprint. A telephone callback or token system can be used to verify the user. Robust firewalls and antivirus protection must be in place. There needs to be a method of electronically blocking unauthorized external access to local area networks, or LANs. One good requirement of access control is to install automatic logoff at workstations. Another good technique to limit access is to disable any unnecessary services running on all the servers, workstations, and even the network itself. Disable all unused protocols and close unused ports. The method for securing workstations is not specified so entities can find the best fit to their particular situation. Some of the questions the security officer must address are these:

- Is the list of approved authorized users maintained and updated regularly?

- Are unauthorized intrusion efforts adequately blocked?

- Are personnel files matched with user accounts to be sure workers who have been terminated or transferred do not retain system access?

- Are passwords changed every 90 days or sooner?

- Are passwords hidden when entered?

- Are passwords stored securely and according to the policy?

- Are passwords automatically offered by an autofill feature?

- Are temporary vendor passwords deleted immediately?

- Does the workstation limit the number of invalid access attempts that may occur for a given user?

- Is only "minimum necessary" allowed?

- Are robust antivirus intrusion measures in place?

Passwords should not be easily guessed. Passwords using pets, names, or dictionary words are easily guessed. They should be a minimum of six (6) characters of mixed upper- and lowercase letters and include numbers. It currently takes a hacker less than a minute to guess any combination of four characters. With current computer speeds, a hacker will take several hours to guess a five-character code and several weeks to guess a six-character code. Good security demands proper usage of passwords and a regular schedule to change them. An industry standard for any business organization expects a change of passwords every 90 days or sooner. The expectation for the Security Rule is no different.

TRUE STORY

A hacker downloaded medical records, health information, and social security numbers on more than 5,000 patients at the University of Washington Medical Center. The hacker was motivated by a desire to expose the vulnerability of electronic medical records. (O'Harrow, 2000).

HIPAA does not require the use of electronic signatures. If a health care provider chooses to move to a paperless environment, then electronic signatures will be necessary. This eliminates further paper added to the medical record but adds to the problem of keeping e-PHI secure. Electronic signatures must provide the combination of authenticity, message integrity, and "nonrepudiation" that is necessary in an electronic environment. **Nonrepudiation** means a method by which the sender of data is provided with proof of delivery and the recipient is assured of the sender's identity, so that neither can later deny having processed the data. Some signatures reproduce the actual written signature as an image and place that on the document through password protection. Other systems require a set of passwords and then print the physician's name, date, time, and the statement "This is electronically signed" to the document. To date, the DHHS has not adopted a standard for electronic signatures. This technology is still evolving. The government is sure that viable solutions will be available soon. Until that time, the electronic signature requirements in the HIPAA ruling are not thoroughly addressed.

Audit Controls

The security standards emphasize the need to train persons about the value of **audit trails** in computerized record systems. An audit trail examines the information system activity to track which password or station accessed information (who: login ID); what information was accessed and what was done to it (read-only, modify, delete, add, etc.); and when (time stamp). Changes to the information are allowed for a limited time. After a specified time, the information entered into the electronic system must become permanent. Only addendums are permitted then. This way there is a record of the original entry, the adjustments to it, and the timing of the change. Some questions to answer are these:

- Does the audit trail support "after-the-fact" investigations of how, when, and why normal operations ceased?

- Is access to online audit logs strictly controlled?

- Is there a separate person in charge of administering access control functions from the person who administers the audit trail?

- Is suspicious activity investigated and appropriate action taken?

- Has the system been thoroughly tested for security?

- When was the last test? It is within a year and documented?

Integrity

The definition of **integrity** of e-PHI means that the entity is required to confirm that data in its possession is accurate and has not been altered, lost, or destroyed in an unauthorized manner. This section of the Security

Rule looks at protection of data from accidental or malicious alteration and destruction. It is designed to provide assurance to the user that the information meets federal expectations about its quality and integrity. The security officer must consider some issues like the following:

- Is virus detection and virus elimination software installed and activated?

- Is any inappropriate or unusual activity reported and investigated, and appropriate action taken?

- Are intrusion detection tools installed on the system?

Clearly many of these items require sophisticated knowledge of information systems and their functions. For this reason, this standard is addressable to meet the needs of the health care provider.

Person or Entity Authorization

Anyone logging on to the electronic system must be identified with login and password. Care must be taken to keep passwords private and change them on a regular basis. Authorization systems must limit the times a user can attempt access if the password is not accurate. **Authentication**, or the confirmation that a person is the one claimed, must be secure and updated as employees move or change responsibilities. The following true story shows how important it is to limit access to *anyone* other than the authorized user.

TRUE STORY

The 13-year-old daughter of a hospital employee took a list of patients' names and phone numbers from the hospital when visiting her mother at work. As a joke, she contacted patients and told them that they were diagnosed with HIV. (The Washington Post, 1995).

Transmission Security

The Security Rule requires protection of health information when being transmitted. The data must be protected in a manner corresponding to the associated risk. This means using **encryption** technology as it is sent over the Internet or dial-up lines. Encryption technology changes readable text into a vast series of "garbled" characters using complex mathematical **algorithms** (a step-by-step procedure for solving a problem). Another way of defining encryption is to use an algorithmic process to transform data into a format in which there is a low probability of assigning meaning to the result without using a confidential process or key. Once encrypted, data can be transmitted over unsecured lines. Because older codes can be easily broken, the encryption technology needs to be reevaluated routinely. With the introduction of wireless devices, like handheld devices, tablet PCs, and notebooks, security through encryption is difficult to achieve. Many software companies are working to improve this technology to bring about security and integrity of data to the wireless devices. Point-to-point communication via a modem is considered to be secure. A virtual private network (VPN) is a point-to-point "tunnel" through the Internet accomplished by a special encryption technique. It is not required that data transmitted through a LAN (local area network) protected from the Internet be encrypted. It is not required to encrypt data *at rest* either. Encryption is left as an addressable issue. The specifics are up to the covered entity to decide.

With electronic claims submission, the computer system must be able to identify the entity that is sending the information as well as who is receiving it. This information is included in the transmission so the software program should refuse receipt by an unauthorized entity. The sending entity must keep track of changes to identifiers so there is not any mix-up with transmissions.

Organization Requirements

The organization requirements focus mainly on the aspect of business associate (BA) contracts. This section also covers certain requirements that health plans must meet. Covered entities are required to have appropriate contracts with all business associates. Within the contract with business associates are provisions stating that all reasonable and appropriate safeguards are in place. The BA is to protect the confidentiality, integrity, and availability of e-PHI that they create, receive, maintain, or transmit. Part of the organization requirements is that any security incident must be documented and reported to the other entity. If violations are found with a particular BA, and reasonable and appropriate corrections are not made promptly, then the covered entity is to terminate the contract with that BA.

Health care clearinghouses process a large portion of the total volume of health claims. They provide a service to providers by filtering claims from many health care providers through their editing system to ensure accuracy. They adjust claims to fit the needs of the various health plans. Then the clearinghouse forwards the claims in large batches to the specific health plans. They act as an intermediary. Thus, each provider does not have to be concerned with the specifics of health plan requirements. These clearinghouses must maintain security of all e-PHI they process just as a health care provider does. The same measures implemented by a health care provider or health plan are to be used and documented by health care clearinghouses. The BA contract between the clearinghouse and the health care provider must state that reasonable and appropriate safeguards are in place to protect the confidentiality, integrity, and availability of the e-PHI they process.

Policies, Procedures, and Documentation

The Security Rule requires that all policies be accessible for review either in electronic policy form or on paper in a location that is readily available to all employees. These policies are to be reviewed on a regular basis to ensure compliance. They must be updated regularly as rulings change. The security officer is to consult the DHHS regularly to see if changes have been posted that affect the health care provider. All documentation of policies and procedures are to be kept for six years even though the wording has changed or been eliminated. This allows an investigator to go back to what a policy said six years ago even though the current policy may read differently. This way if an incident is under investigation, documentation is available to see what steps were in force at the time of the incident.

IMPACT ON ORGANIZATIONS

Physicians' offices and clinics face the challenge to continue business without interruption to patients while maintaining procedures to comply with HIPAA. Where the physician practice is small, the burden of compliance falls on a very limited number of workers. Entities may not have money available to readily purchase equipment and technical assistance to comply. The DHHS sees HIPAA compliance as a pathway. However, the department is expecting covered entities to have completed the steps to compliance. The federal government understands that security cannot be perfect. It allows for the "reasonableness" of protections. The security officer might consider the comical example of two hunters being chased by a bear. One hunter is just making sure he can outrun the other guy. Much of the same concept is true of security protections for electronic data. Strive to be more secure than most other organizations. That way you are not as likely to be a target or be audited by federal investigators.

Many hospitals have come up against a budget shortfall. There are cutbacks in federal reimbursements. Private health plans have revised their payments and lowered reimbursements too. Insurance coverage of prescriptions has had to balance the increasing use of medications and their increasing cost against maintaining premiums that individuals can afford. It is hard for many hospitals to provide funds to cover the costs of the standards. The DHHS has purposely written the standards to be "technology neutral." No one product has the only answer to the security requirements. Yet the challenge is to build a technology base and infrastructure that will be able to grow and continue to meet the requirements.

A technology that is becoming increasing utilized is telemedicine. Telemedicine is using videoconferencing to conduct an office visit with a physician located at a distant location. Many hospitals, both large and small, are becoming involved with this means of conducting patient encounters. This is referred to as an *interactive videoconferencing consultation*. Using the Internet, a patient can have an office visit with a physician located many miles away. The patient is monitored at the site locally, and health information may be transmitted to the consulting physician along with the visual image. The consulting physician can watch the patient move, walk, or perform other activity just as if he or she were in the room. Generally, a physician's assistant is on site to conduct any tests or procedures the consulting doctor may request. The discussion between patient and physician via videoconferencing brings both parties together so well that the idea of distance is forgotten. It can seem as if the doctor and patient are actually in the same location. Often these consultations are videotaped so either the consulting physician or the local provider can review the interview and provide their report. The DHHS has submitted the following definition for security of these videotapes. The videotapes themselves are not part of the medical record and should be erased after standard documentation of care is complete. The patient must provide written consent before the taping. Written consent may be omitted if documentation relates to abuse or neglect. Under usual circumstances, the videotape would be erased shortly after the encounter, and the only record of the teleconference would be the electronic or paper report with the physician's signature. The physician's report is to include the final disposition of the videotape, whether it was erased, or if not erased, where it will be kept. (Telehealth Update, 2000). Tapes may be kept that have educational value to medical students. If any educational tapes are retained, they are not to have any personal identifiers. They must be de-identified as specified under the HIPAA Privacy Rule.

CHALLENGES TO COMPLIANCE AND ENFORCEMENT

The DHHS has written Security Rules in a manner that applies to any size of organization. The challenge is to see greater efficiency in the process of paying the provider for health care, and at the same time reduce the cost involved with doing business. Many entities have seen an initial cost involved to change hardware and software systems. As the implementation continues, the return on the investment will grow. This will happen through simplifying the administration of claims. The time needed to process health claims will decrease.

The federal government understands that it is impossible to keep e-PHI totally secure. The goal of DHHS is to see documentation that the covered entity, whether a health care provider, health care clearinghouse, or health plan, has taken steps to ensure the safety and security of e-PHI. This means a balance must be struck between the identifiable risks and the cost of protective measures. As with the Privacy Rule, the rule of thumb is to provide reasonable and appropriate security for the particular situation the covered entity finds. The risk analysis and risk management plan are basic to compliance. These risk documents are to be part of the documentation maintained by the security officer. The challenge to managing the security process comes in funding the necessary changes plus finding people and resources qualified to bring about the changes required.

A typical hospital workforce includes both paid and nonemployee workers (physicians), making enforcement of security standards more challenging. Many hospitals utilize a large number of volunteer workers to perform routine and hospital responsibilities. Including volunteer workers in the workforce adds another challenge to manage security for them as well.

The day-to-day access to the health care facility must be protected. At the same time, visitors and those with physical handicaps should not be hindered from gaining entrance and exit. Doors need to be monitored to reduce the risk of theft or unintended disclosure of information. The security officer needs to balance the risk of the particular situation with the cost to prevent unauthorized access to health information.

A big challenge in keeping transmissions secure is the increasing use of Internet communication. Most Internet-based e-mail is not sent in an encrypted format. PHI is not to be e-mailed unless a security algorithm is in place. More and better wireless technology is available and requires special attention to keep information secure.

For covered entities wishing to file a complaint of noncompliance, there are two ways to file. The CMS web site, http://www.cms.hhs.gov, has a link to a downloadable form. This is mailed to the Office of E-Health Standards and Services (OESS). The other is by Internet using the Administrative Simplification Enforcement Tool (ASET), currently located at http://www.cms.hhs.gov; search for ASET. These are to be used by covered entities only as a last resort to resolve compliance issues with a trading partner or a business associate. The OESS operates as a separate entity under CMS and is completely detached from CMS's Medicare- and Medicaid-related activities. The Office of HIPAA Standards (OHS) is a separate division of the DHHS. This office is responsible for enforcement of the Security Rule. The OESS receives complaints, then passes them to the appropriate enforcement agency, in this case the OHS. As with Privacy Rule compliance, CMS is looking for voluntary

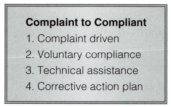

FIGURE 4-1 Steps to move toward compliance with HIPAA

compliance and reasonable diligence to correct problems encountered. Figure 4-1 lists steps to move from complaint to compliance.

Stanley Nachimson, senior technical advisor of the Office for HIPAA Standards, outlined steps his office views essential toward bringing compliance to covered entities. (Nachimson, 2005).

Any covered entity that follows these steps would find assistance and help from the government office. If an accused covered entity does not respond to CMS, fines could be imposed as a last resort. Filing a complaint with OHS should only be considered after working with a trading partner to resolve a dispute. Complaints will be classified as to severity and handled individually. The office will maintain the anonymity of the filer as much as possible. (Trudel, 2004). Though the OHS will investigate complaints, they have also chosen to begin audits of certain facilities where compliance may be lacking. If compliance is not forthcoming, the OHS may levy fines of not more than $100 per violation or $25,000 per calendar year for violations of identical requirements or prohibitions. The DHHS has authority to assess the civil monetary penalties. The Department of Justice has the authority to prosecute criminal penalties. Further discussion is included in Chapter 5 of this book. "Unique Health Identifiers and HIPAA Myths."

Summary

The HIPAA Security Rule covers any protected health information that is in electronic form. This may be information that is transmitted or "at rest." "At rest" may be at an off-site facility as backup. The Privacy Rule protects health information from being used or disclosed in ways that are not authorized unless for means of treatment, payment, or normal health care business operations. The Security Rule expects that health information be kept protected. Procedures must be in place to maintain the integrity of the data within information systems. Access to necessary information is to be available to those authorized to view the health information. Security includes protection against anticipated threats or hazards. In order to comply with the federal ruling, each covered entity must consider five main areas of compliance.

1. Administrative safeguards
2. Physical safeguards
3. Technical safeguards
4. Organization requirements
5. Policy and procedure documentation

The administration of each entity must analyze the risks within their organization with a *risk analysis*. Then, it must develop a plan to minimize those risks of unauthorized disclosure or access to the electronic health information they maintain with a *risk management plan*. One specific person is to be designated as *security officer*. This officer may oversee a committee, depending upon the size of the entity. Each person on the workforce must be trained in use of security measures to access the information needed to perform his or her job. The information access is limited to the "minimum necessary" as explained in the Privacy Rule. If any attempted or successful security incident is found, the incident is to be documented and steps taken to remedy the situation immediately. Each covered entity must have written *continuity plans* in case of disaster of any kind. The Security Rule expects to find periodic evaluation of the safeguards to measure their effectiveness. All BA contracts must have addition information to safeguard e-PHI the BA may encounter in the course of business.

The physical security of the building, electronic storage equipment, and workstations is the focus of the second portion of the Security Rule. *Access* to locations where protected health information is stored must be secure. All *workstations* must be located to maximize security, and software logoff timers must be in place to minimize unauthorized access. Any electronic device, whether stationary or portable, containing e-PHI must be logged, especially when it is taken out of service. The security officer is expected to oversee that information held within these devices is erased, deleted, or destroyed appropriately.

Within the management of electronic equipment, there must be controls to the levels of access dependent upon the job description. An *audit trail* must be present to trace data movement and access. *Authentication* must be secure and updated as employees move or change responsibilities. Under the technical safeguards, the transmission of e-PHI must be kept secure through *encryption* methods.

As of 2003, there were an estimated 4 million plus health plans and another 1.2 million plus health care providers, besides many health care clearinghouses, which facilitate claims between the providers and payers.

Many of these entities have moved to an electronic system because continuing with paper forms was so much more costly in time and storage than the cost of storing and transmitting health information electronically. In fact, the change from paper to electronic storage was effectively mandated. Almost all claims are now processed electronically. The Security Rule of HIPAA will not apply to the covered entity if it is totally paper-based. However, if *any* of its information is kept or transmitted in electronic format, then the Security Rule must be adopted with appropriate policies and procedures implemented to ensure compliance.

REVIEW QUESTIONS

1. A covered entity must comply with the Security Rule if _____ protected health information (PHI) is kept or transmitted.

2. Give examples of information not covered by the Security Rule.

3. The Privacy Rule covers keeping PHI private. What type of PHI does the Security Rule address? Does this overlap with the Privacy Rule? In what way does it overlap?

4. Summarize unique responsibilities of the security officer in various facilities.

5. Discuss some risks that may be found in maintaining security of PHI within a physician's office, freestanding clinic, ambulatory surgical center, long-term care facility, inpatient rehabilitation facility, pathology lab, pharmacy, and durable medical equipment store.

6. Match definitions with words.

   a) Security incident

   b) Risk analysis

   c) Continuity plan

   d) Clearinghouse

      i. _____A process whereby cost-effective security and control measures may be selected by balancing the cost of various security and control measures against the losses that would be expected if these measures were not in place

      ii. _____A plan including applications and data criticality analysis, a data backup plan, a disaster recovery plan, an emergency mode operation plan, and testing and revision procedures

      iii. _____The attempted or successful unauthorized access, use, disclosure, modification, or destruction of information or interference with system operations in an information system

iv. _____Receives a standard transaction from another entity and processes or facilitates the processing of information into nonstandard format or nonstandard data content for a receiving entity

7. Discuss password protection and the need for privacy of passwords for each workstation at a health care facility. Remembering passwords is problematic for some people. Why is it so essential?

8. Consider physical access to facilities—ease of access is to be given patients, yet how could that allow for unauthorized entrance?

9. Discuss some issues about security that would be easy to try to compromise.

10. Since some items under the Security Rule are "addressable," does this allow the security office to document that the standard cannot be followed? What measures are permitted?

11. In the spring, many workplaces have encouraged parents to bring their child to work with them to experience a parent's day. What precautions relating to HIPAA must be implemented when visitors like children visit a facility?

12. Any security incident must be disclosed to the individuals involved. Consider the impact on a health care facility when the access is to their database and perhaps thousands of patient records have been exposed. How is the facility to manage this breach within HIPAA rules?

References

Briggs, B. (2004, March). Taming the infrastructure beast. *Health Data Management*, 12-3, 37.

CA appellate court says plaintiff's signed release bars HIV privacy suit. (2000, February 22). *AIDS Litigation Reporter*.

DHS surplus sales again reveal confidential information, (2002, April). Associated Press.

Ernst & Young. (2003, August 22). Advancing health in America. *Regulatory Advisory*, p. 2.

Estate of Behringer v. Medical Center at Princeton, 249 NJ Super. 507 (1991).

Health Insurance Reform: Security Standards; Final Rule, 68 Fed. Reg. 8,333–8,381 (February 20, 2003) (to codify 45 C.F.R. parts 160, 162, and 164).

Nachimson, S. Office of HIPAA Standards, *HIPAA Administrative Simplification Standards Yesterday, Today, and Tomorrow*. CMS. Presentation at the CMS Atlanta Regional 2005 Provider Session. February 10, 2005.

Notice of Proposed Rule Making (NPRM): Security and Electronic Signature Standards. (last modified January 31, 2003). Centers for Medicare and Medicaid Services. Retrieved September 17, 2003, from http://www.cms.hhs.gov/hipaa/hipaa2/regulations/security/nprm/sec11.asp.

O'Harrow, R. (2000, December 9). Hacker accesses patient records. *Washington Post*, p. E1.

Telehealth Update, Office for the Advancement of Telemedicine. (February 18, 2000). Retrieved September 17, 2003, from http://telehealth.hrsa.gov/pubs/privac/htm.

The 13-year-old daughter of a hospital employee. *Washington Post*, 1 March 1995.

Trudel, K, Acting Director of Office of HIPAA Standards. (2004, March 8). *Where We Are Now, Where We Are Going*. Presented at the HIPAA Standards 8th National HIPAA Summit.

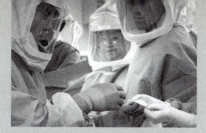

CHAPTER
5

UNIQUE HEALTH IDENTIFIERS AND HIPAA MYTHS

OBJECTIVES

Identify the unique identifiers defined by HIPAA.

Recognize which identifiers have been mandated and the status of other identifiers to date.

Know where to find the latest information on changes to HIPAA law.

Explain the problem of medical identify theft.

Dispel some myths related to HIPAA.

KEY TERMS

check digit

employer identification number (EIN)

national provider identifier (NPI)

medical identity theft

INTRODUCTION

T*he HIPAA law authorizes the Department of Health and Human Services (DHHS) to develop unique identifiers for all parties included in a health claim. The entities included are the following:*

1. *Health care providers*
2. *Health plans*
3. *Employers*
4. *Patients*

This portion of HIPAA law has been implemented in stages. The first and easiest identifiers to standardize were the employer numbers. The next standardized identifier developed was the health care provider. After that came the health plan unique identifier. Finally will come the individual patient identifier, if the DHHS will receive authority to develop it.

We will summarize the focus of the HIPAA law, since sometimes it is hard to remember the big picture. It is easy to get lost in details. The health care industry is now faced with possible civil and criminal charges if either the privacy of health information is violated or security of the protected health information is breached in an unauthorized manner. All health care professionals need to be aware of the consequences of any action that is in violation of this federal law. Also, as the health care industry has wrestled with the rules, misconceptions have developed about what HIPAA does permit and does not permit. Lastly, we will explore some of the most common myths that have arisen about HIPAA.

THINK ABOUT IT

1. Identification numbers help keep covered entities clearly identified, but are the names not just as good an identifier?
2. People have enough numbers to remember now. Do we need more? Would the inclusion of these new numbers eliminate others?
3. How would national provider identifiers help simplify anything?
4. What are the issues surrounding and delaying individual health identifiers?

REASONS FOR IDENTIFICATION NUMBERS

Participants in the delivery of health care and health care payments include health care providers, health plans, employers, and the individuals receiving care. By standardizing health care transactions into codes rather than lengthy explanations or nonuniform names, the DHHS has greatly streamlined the transmission and processing of transactions. This allows more information to be processed in a shorter time frame than if printed and mailed to the health plan. The codes bring a desirable efficiency. The last step in the Health Insurance Portability and Accountability Act of 1996 (HIPAA) is to uniformly identify the participants within the transaction according to a federal standard. This simplification eliminates possible confusion of identity and removes distinctions between covered entities and employers. The law was written to require unique identifiers for all parties included in health care claims. At the time of this writing, the DHHS had developed the final rule requiring unique identifiers for health care providers. Unique identifiers for health plans will follow. Originally, the law included the development of unique health identifiers for individuals. The DHHS and Congress currently have postponed the development of the individual identifiers due to strong public resistance. (Fact Sheet, Administrative Simplification under HIPAA, 2003). There are some options for unique identifiers that will possibly be considered.

Several organizations have been involved in determining the identifier standards to be adopted. These organizations are mentioned in the legislation. The important considerations are that the standard must improve the efficiency, effectiveness, and safety of the health care system. The standard must meet the needs of the health data user community. The code system must be consistent and uniform with other HIPAA standards in providing privacy and security.

Employer Identifier

The DHHS standardized employer identifiers first. When identifying an employer in a standard transaction as defined under the HIPAA Transaction and Code Set Ruling, the standard unique employer identifier (SUEI) must be used. This identifier is not required for most claim forms generated by the health care provider. The need for an employer identification number in a health care claim would be in the following transactions:

1. ASC X12N 834—Benefit Enrollment and Maintenance

2. ASC X12N 270/271—Health Care Eligibility Benefit Inquiry and Response

3. ASC X12N 820—Health Plan Premium Payments

4. ASC X12N 837—Health Care Claim: Dental, Professional, or Institutional

The DHHS defined this identifier to be the employer identification number (EIN) issued by the Internal Revenue Service (IRS) under the authority of the Department of the Treasury. This standard was adopted after consultation with several organizations responsible for developing the transaction standards. They include the National Uniform Billing Committee (NUBC), the National Uniform Claim Committee (NUCC), the Workgroup for Electronic Data Interchange (WEDI), and the American Dental Association (ADA). The specific focus of these groups was explained in chapter 3, "Transactions and Code Sets."

The DHHS issued the final rule regarding SUEI in July 2002. The rule focused on employers. The employer of a patient or a patient's dependent was made responsible to ensure enrollment status in the employer's particular health plan. The standard adopted is the EIN. Those small employers who provide health care coverage and use a social security number (SSN) as their tax identification number (TIN) must secure an EIN for use in the electronic transactions.

The **employer identification number (EIN)** is a nine-digit code with a hyphen after the second digit: 00-0000000. This is the number that appears on the IRS Form W-2, Wage and Tax Statement, and appears on the employee's tax form. The IRS defined the format of two digits, a hyphen, and seven more digits. The first two digits of the employer identification number reflect the issuing Internal Revenue district. The rest of the numbers are unique identifiers with no "intelligence," that is, there is no formatting to indicate more information about a specific employer. In the final rule, the DHHS authorized the use of the hyphen within the number. This is contrary to optical character reader guidelines that eliminate all punctuation so the reader does not misinterpret information. Because most employers already had an employer identification number, the shift to adoption for HIPAA was relatively easy. (Health Insurance Reform, 2002).

The use of this identifier is *required* when used between health plans and employers enrolling and disenrolling in a health plan. This is when an ASC X12N 834—Benefit Enrollment and Maintenance in a Health Plan—transaction is used. This transaction identifies the sponsor of the health plan when the sponsor is a self-insured employer. Other uses of the EIN are *situational*—depending on if the unique employer must be identified. Most uses do not involve the health care provider.

Presently, there are five *situational* uses of the standard unique employer identifier in electronic transactions.

1. X12N 270/271—Health Care Eligibility Benefit Inquiry and Response. Generally the health plan and employer communicate this information, and the health care provider is not involved. The information is to verify that an employee is participating in the employer's group health plan. It is not PHI so HIPAA law does not apply.

2. X12N 276/277—Health Care Claim Status Request/Response. Employers identify themselves as the source of information about eligibility of individuals in a workers' compensation claim. This is a situational use because the employer is not a covered entity and e-PHI is not transmitted. Most health care providers will have a relationship with the employer to treat workers' compensation cases and already know the EIN.

3. X12N 834—Benefit Enrollment and Maintenance in a Health Plan. Use of the EIN is *situational* when used to identify the employer of a person covered under a health plan when that employer is *not* the sponsor. This differs from the *required* use explained above.

4. X12N 820—Health Plan Premium Payments. Employers use their EIN to identify themselves in transactions when enrolling or disenrolling their employees in a health plan. This transaction is not mentioned in chapter 3, "Transactions and Code Sets," since this does not involve the health care provider.

5. ASC X12N 837—Health Care Claim: Dental, Professional, or Institutional. Use of these transactions for workers' compensation claims at present is still being developed by the DHHS.

The compliance date for all covered entities was August 2005. Enforcement of this ruling is under the direction of the Office for HIPAA Standards (OHS) under CMS.

Health Care Provider Identifier

All health care providers had at least one identifier. Many providers had several. Medicare issued a number and Medicaid organizations issued another. Health plans often issued their own identifier to be used on their claims. The national provider identifier (NPI) as developed by the Centers for Medicare and Medicaid Service (CMS) is *replacing all of these currently used identifiers*. The unique physician identification numbers (UPIN) contained "intelligence," meaning that information can be determined just by knowing the position format of the code. These identifiers also contain "intelligence" about entity. Licensed pharmacies were assigned a seven-digit identifier by the National Association of Boards of Pharmacy (NABP). This identifier had "intelligence" embedded in the code identifying the state where the pharmacy is located. Many health care providers were issued a different number, the NPI. The HIPAA ruling has the same name *but is not the same identifier*. Every health care provider must apply for a NPI number through the National Provider System under the HIPAA regulations.

The DHHS has had input from many organizations to define the best identifier for providers of health care. The final rule was issued January 2004 and was effective May 2004. The NUBC, which oversees hospital billing forms such as UB-92 and the new UB-04, has had input into the adoption. Also the ADA, the NUCC (the group that reviews changes to the provider insurance claims on CMS-1500 and the new CMS-2004), and the Workgroup for Electronic Data Interchange (WEDI) have sent recommendations to the secretary of DHHS. They find that the NPI maintained by the CMS fits the requirements listed above.

The **national provider identifier (NPI)** is a 10-digit number system with the last digit being a **check digit**. A check digit provides a means to check that the number is accurate. An algorithm sums the nine digits and uses the digit on the right or the "ones" column number as the check. If numbers are transposed or entered in error, the check digit will not match and an error will be spotted. The International Standards Organization (ISO), which certifies many international and national businesses, uses the check digit in many standardized transactions. The NPI contains no embedded information about the provider that could identify the entity. The identifier will be able to accommodate all types of health care providers, for example, physicians, hospitals, license practitioners, suppliers of medical equipment, group practices, pharmacies, and certain noninstitutional providers such as ambulance companies. The CMS believes that any identifier adopted must be capable of at least 100 million unique identifiers. This system is estimated to meet the needs of our country for about 200 years. CMS has defined two categories of health care providers for enumeration purposes.

- Entity Type Code 1 is issued to providers who are individual human beings.

- Entity Type Code 2 is designated for providers other than individuals, that is, organizations.

For billing purposes, it is vital to know the proper NPI to submit on a claim since many providers may be part of an organization as well as have obtained their own personal NPI. (HIPAA Administrative Simplification, 2004). The deadline for compliance was May 23, 2007, and small health plans have an additional year, until May 23, 2008, in order to comply. (HIPAA Administrative Simplification, 2004). Note that health plans are the *insurance* providers, not the health care providers who have another year for compliance.

Health Plan Identifier

Each health plan will also have a unique identifier to go along with the identifiers for each health care provider and employer that uses standardized transactions. The development of this standard is under the direction of the same committees that designated the standards for employers and providers of health care. The unique identifier for health plans is suggested to be the same as for employers (the EIN), but the DHHS has not made any official decision as of this writing. A proposed ruling by the DHHS is expected in the near future.

Personal Identifier

Several organizations have begun to develop systems to identify individuals. The idea of a national identifier for each individual who may visit an institution for some type of health care is quite controversial. There are many ramifications to issuing every person in the United States a unique identification number. The very idea hints at invasion of personal privacy by governmental organizations to an even greater degree than some people imagine currently exists. Imagine the many entities that might have health information about one patient—a primary care physician, several specialists, anesthesiologist, laboratory, hospital, pharmacist, durable medical equipment supplier, clinic, and mail-order prescription provider—just to treat one ailment. If records were to be interconnected through electronic medical records (EMR), each of these providers would be linked to the one personal identifier.

There are two very good reasons to have individual identifiers.

1. The quality of health care would be enhanced since there would be an accurate and rapid identification of an individual's health record spanning all providers.

2. With one coordinated location for all health information, physicians would be able to coordinate medications prescribed by other providers and avoid allergic reactions to drugs and adverse drug interactions. (Davidson and Holtz, 1998).

Concerns against a personal identifier include the following:

1. Confidentiality and privacy intrusions

2. Choice of the individual identifier—that it is truly unique

3. Legal protection of the information

4. The costs associated with moving to a new identifier

5. Who should pay for the costs of the transition

6. Issues dealing with accurate implementation of patient records by all entities (Identifiers, 2004)

7. How do individuals keep accurate record of their number?

8. Ease of identity theft

Even though legislation originally mandated this type of identifier, plans for implementation by the DHHS are at a standstill. The DHHS has published a white paper and has opened up the opportunity for discussion of this issue. Public comment has been encouraged. The DHHS is waiting for approval before developing unique health identifiers for individuals.

Several organizations are developing plans to establish a unique identifier for patients for possible future use. (Unique Identifiers, 2004). Here is information about seven possible systems that could be considered.

1. Standard guide for properties of a universal health identifier (UHID)

2. Social security number (SSN)

3. Biometrics ID

4. Directory service

5. Personal immutable properties

6. Patient identification system based on existing medical record number and practitioner prefix

7. Public key—private key cryptology method

The current practice of identifying an individual consists of a medical record number or alphanumeric code issued by the individual provider organization. This is unique to the entity and not transferable to other systems. Some software vendors have explored developing a means to use these medical record numbers combined with a provider number to come up with a corporate master patient index. This system does not have much validity to be nationalized. The other identification systems listed above have more potential should the DHHS choose to adopt a standard. We will summarize each system.

Standard guide for properties of a universal health identifier (UHID) is a standard being developed by the American Society for Testing and Materials (ASTM). The scheme of the identifier consists of a sequential identifier, a delimiter, check digits, and an encryption scheme to support data security. This system allows for automatically linking to various computer-based records. It supports data security of privileged clinical information and uses technology to keep operating cost to a minimum. It is reported that two veterans, hospitals are now implementing this system.

A *social security number (SSN)* was originally planned to function only for the Social Security Administration. It has become a personal identifier with many applications, including use by local, state, and federal authorities; financial institutions; and many consumer organizations. There are a number of issues that disqualify this system from being sufficient. These issues are the following:

- Social security numbers are not entirely unique.
- They lack check digits.
- There is a significant error rate.
- There are privacy and confidentiality risks.
- They lack legal protection and capacity for future growth.
- They lack a mechanism for emergency use.
- There is no provision for noncitizens.

The Computer-based Record Institute (CPRI) is exploring using a modified social security number to include check digits and an encryption scheme.

Biometrics ID may use fingerprint, retinal pattern analysis, voice pattern identification, and DNA analysis as possible identifiers. There are law enforcement and immigration departments who use some of the biometric identification methods already. At present, there are no standards, procedures, or guidelines for this type of use in the health care industry. Concerns for this identification system relate to organ transplant, amputation, and diseases affecting organs used for identification such as retinopathy affecting retinal pattern analysis.

A *directory service* is a proposal being developed by the Mitre Corporation. The Mitre Corporation is working to provide linkages with existing patient identifiers to allow connections across computer systems. They propose including social characteristics such as name, social security number, address, driver's license, etc., with physical characteristics like fingerprint or retina scans. They propose using these along with other groupings such as gender, race, and identification data at the current point of care. By connecting all of these identifiers electronically to other point-of-care locations, information could be exchanged with a great accuracy. This is only being explored and is not in practice anywhere. Costs to implement this type of identification would be considerable.

Physicians at the Mayo Clinic are considering *personal immutable properties*. Their proposal consists of a series of three universal immutable values plus a check digit. The three values are a seven-digit date of birth field, a six-digit place of birth code, a five-digit sequence code (to separate individuals born on the same date in the same geographic area), and a single check digit. This would be called a unique patient identifier (UPI).

Patient identification system based on existing medical record number and practitioner prefix is a system proposed by the Medical Records

TABLE 5-1   Table of Identifiers

Entity	Acronym	Name	Implementation Date
Employer	EIN	Employer Identification Number	2004
Health Care Provider	NPI	National Provider Identifier	2007
Health Plan			Under development
Patient			None foreseen

Institute. This patient identification number uses the provider institution's patient medical record number with a provider number as prefix. This use of already-defined numbers eliminates the cost of creating a new patient numbering system. The unique provider number would identify the location of the patient database, and the medical record number would identify the patient's record within that database. This system allows the patient to designate a practitioner of choice to be the curator or gateway to connect other data systems and update information.

The *public key—private key cryptography method* is a method being proposed by a doctor working with the Massachusetts Institute of Technology. This system of identifiers uses smart cards or keys and computers for accessing patient information. Two keys would be necessary to allow arbitrary messages to be encoded and decoded. The two keys would contain mathematical functions that are inverse to each other. One key is a patient private key. The other is an organizational/provider key. Together they generate and maintain identifiers that are specific and unique to the organization and individual patients within that organization. An umbrella organization would handle the patient private keys via an ID server. The patient will have the public key of the organization. With this concept, outside organizations requesting information would only gain access with the private key of the patient. This plan relies heavily on computer technology.

These are possible solutions to the unique health identifiers as directed in the HIPAA law of 1996.

WHAT IS IMPORTANT TO KNOW ABOUT HIPAA?

Congress directed the DHHS to write rules mandating that all providers of health care, all health plans, and all health care clearinghouses

1. adhere to a uniform set of standards to *ensure the privacy* of an individual's health care information

2. make it *easier for people* who move to another job *to continue or begin health insurance coverage*

3. *standardize electronic transactions* by developing code sets and identifiers to be used

4. keep the electronic data containing *health information secure from adverse events or a breach in security.*

Efficiency and uniformity have been the goal of the Title II rulings. That is the reason for calling it "Administrative Simplification." This causes changes to varying degrees for the covered entities involved. Facilities who handle data electronically within their organization are realizing savings in turnaround time to receive payment for services, increased revenue from more efficient methods of conducting business, and greater patient confidence that the provider will have their best interests in mind. The DHHS will need to modify their rules to adjust to new challenges. The department has promised this will happen. Any rule will stand for at least 24 months. It may be modified after that, as seems necessary. Those responsible for compliance such as the HIPAA officer need to routinely check with the DHHS's Web site or other government sources to maintain compliance. Refinements are already being issued. Access to the department's Web site is a necessary part of the HIPAA officer's job.

Locating the Latest Title II Rules and Changes

One responsibility of the HIPAA officer is keeping abreast of any changes in the ruling. Medical journals and periodicals are important sources of information. Perhaps the best way to keep up to date is to use the several Web sites under the DHHS. The following are Web sites that will provide good sources of information. It is possible to be on a listserv to receive updates and e-mail notices of changes.

1. The DHHS Web site will have links to HIPAA information at http://www.hhs.gov. This site gives anyone the opportunity to ask questions concerning the rulings. Many questions with their official answers are already posted at this site. Search the Frequently Asked Questions (FAQ) section by topic to see if the question has already been asked

2. At the CMS Web site, http://www.cms.hhs.gov/, search HIPAA links. This is a government site focusing on Medicare and Medicaid services and other health issues. The Office for HIPAA Standards is where complaints concerning nonprivacy violations are submitted. This is under CMS direction. It is an authoritative source of HIPAA information. See Appendix B and C for copies of the fact sheets and complaint forms.

3. Subscribe to the HIPAA REGS listserv for notification via e-mail of all postings on the final rules at http://www.cms.hhs.gov. Search for "listserv." Anyone can enroll in several notification services to receive e-mails of events and changes in federal regulations.

4. See the Government Printing Office for *Federal Register* documents and original source documents, http://www.gpoaccess.gov/. These documents can be long and confusing. The complete *Congressional Record* can be accessed here. Summaries are also available.

5. HIPAA guidelines from the OCR are within the DHHS, http://www.hhs.gov/ocr. The OCR is given the responsibility to oversee compliance with of the HIPAA Privacy Rule.

6. Besides Web sites, current information can be obtained by phoning the Centers for Medicare and Medicaid Services HIPAA HOTLINE: 1-866-282-0659 (Electronic Transactions and Code Sets, 2003)

Appendix B has a listing of the Centers for Medicare and Medicaid Services Regional Offices as well as other resources. A number of health organizations conduct seminars to help interpret rulings and any changes that come along. Local seminars help health care personnel connect with others in the health care field. Networking and sharing of ideas with other health care providers is another valuable source of ideas.

Legal Ramifications of HIPAA

Enough time has elapsed since HIPAA became enforceable law that court cases have begun to appear. As of this writing, decisions in three prominent cases involving HIPAA enforcement have begun to establish precedence. According to NewsBank, quoting the *Fort Worth Star-Telegram* (Texas), 19,240 grievances have been lodged nationwide as of June 5, 2006. More than 73 percent (more than 14,000) of the grievances have been closed either by ruling that there was no violation or by allowing accused entities to promise better compliance. Of the 5,000 remaining cases as of 2006, 309 have been referred to the Department of Justice as possible criminal violations. (Stein, 2007).

HIPAA was written to apply to covered entities, causing them as organizations to sustain liability for noncompliance. HIPAA is quite clear that any alleged violations are to be reported to DHHS via a complaint process. The authors of HIPAA, and Congress, who passed the law, did not intend HIPAA to be the basis for a plaintiff to pursue covered entities directly. In fact, they expressly forbade it. HIPAA law gave the job of enforcement to the DHHS. The secretary of the DHHS, acting through the Office of Inspector General (OIG), established a new health care fraud and abuse control program. Funding is provided through HIPAA allocations. This includes the authority to impose fines and refer possible criminal violations to the Department of Justice. DHHS has designated OCR to investigate all complaints from alleged violations of the Privacy Rule. Allegations in reference to HIPAA privacy complaints are directed to the OCR under the DHHS. (See Appendix B for copy of the privacy complaint form and Appendix C for a copy of the non-privacy complaint form, or access them on the DHHS Web site: http://www.hhs.gov.) The Office of E-Health Services and Standards, not the court system, is the clearinghouse for complaint resolution of nonprivacy complaints. This is the path for allegations from individuals or parties who feel the privacy or security of protected health information has been breached. When either of these offices finds an unwillingness to comply and possible criminal violations, they refer the case to the Department of Justice. On the other side, the OIG, being given the authority to oversee security compliance under HIPAA, can initiate audits of providers for security compliance. This type of investigation is initiated by the DHHS rather than individuals who complain, as in the following example. A hospital in Georgia was targeted for an unannounced audit. This investigation is said to focus on the administrative, physical, and technical safeguards for e-PHI. This is one example of audits initiated by the government rather than complaint driven. More unannounced audits are sure to follow. With the introduction of more technology using wireless connections and other portable devices, it is very important to be thorough ensuring e-PHI is secure. (OIG Launches Audits of Provider Compliance with HIPAA Security Rule, 2007).

A Texas newspaper also quotes Winston Wilkinson, head of the Office of Civil Rights, as saying "Our first approach to dealing with any complaint is to work for voluntary compliance. So far, it's worked out pretty well." (Stein, 2007). This is consistent with earlier comments about enforcement plans attributed to DHHS and accounts for the quick dispatch of so many grievances, as noted above.

It appears that most entities have taken the actions required for compliance. The American Health Information Management Association asked members to report problems they found as they developed policies and procedures for HIPAA. The most common problems appear to be lack of standardized processes for release of PHI and public access to records. Other common problems are the following:

1. Accounting for release of PHI

2. Obtaining PHI from other providers

3. Access and release of information to relatives or spouses

4. Complying with BA provisions

5. Confusion by individuals regarding the Notice of Privacy Practices

6. Access and release of information to law enforcement (Most AHIMA Respondents Say HIPAA Uncovered "Problem Areas," 2004)

From delcotimes.com, there was considerable reference to law enforcement encountering problems with organizations that were overenthusiastic and apparently not well informed about HIPAA compliance. (Mengers, 2004). It has always been the case that appropriate court authority is required before health information may legitimately be released to law enforcement. HIPAA does not interfere with that longstanding situation. Court authority to release information trumps HIPAA and any health care provider policy. HIPAA actually makes it easier for law enforcement to obtain information when there has been criminal activity associated with the health condition of a patient.

It should be noted that medical identity theft or health care services theft is not directly addressed by HIPAA. **Medical identity theft** is defined as "obtaining by theft or deception of personal medical information, such as one's address, social security number, or health insurance information, for use in submitting false claims or seeking medical care or goods." The Federal Trade Commission has logged over 19,000 complaints involving medical identity theft since 1992. Many more thousands of people probably have been affected by theft but are not aware of it or have not reported it. The federal government is moving towards digitizing all medical information to improve health care, reduce fraud, reduce medical errors, and save lives. However, this opens substantial problems from the information technology standpoint to safeguard that digital information from unauthorized access. (Long, 2007). Medical identity theft is covered by other civil and criminal codes that predate HIPAA. However, a health care provider who is compliant with HIPAA is expected to have protection from such thievery, if for no other reason than awareness. It is prudent for an organization to consider risks of identity and health care services theft as separate items and take appropriate action.

One very negative consequence of health care services theft is the damage left behind on the medical record. Similar damage to the permanent record can occur through errors within the health care provider itself. It is surprisingly easy to fraudulently receive medical care. Suppose someone comes by enough information to steal health care services. Presenting at an ER with an injury, a "disoriented" patient offers false information that seems legitimate. To enhance legitimacy, the patient may call upon an accomplice to confirm the stolen credentials as his or her own. All one needs is the name of an employer and perhaps the group number. Claiming a change of address if questioned, the thief allows registration clerks to fill in the rest from existing records, including the medical record number from a previous visit (of the victim). Care is administered and recorded against that permanent record, and only an astute caregiver familiar with the victim might question something slightly amiss. Consider what happens when the victim later presents with a legitimate claim and is treated based upon the medical history of the thief!

Myths about HIPAA

With new rules come many ideas about what they really mean. Since spring of 2003, many rumors have circulated about what the HIPAA law really says and what it does not say. We will explain a few common misconceptions and how compliance with HIPAA really works. Also note that the acronym is not "HIPPA," as in hippopotamus. This is the image many people have when first considering the extent of the HIPAA ruling—that it is as large and bulky as a hippopotamus.

A. *Myth—Appointment reminders:* To protect the privacy of PHI, many receptionists were very concerned about leaving a voice mail reminder of a doctor's appointment. Any information that might be heard by someone other than the patient was a likely unauthorized disclosure. Some offices stopped phoning their patients completely. Some stopped sending postcard reminders. Others did not change procedures at all, hoping nothing would be said.

   Proper response: All information is to be kept to the "minimum necessary" as outlined in the Privacy Rule. There is nothing wrong with leaving voice mail to remind patients of an upcoming appointment. Date, time, and the name of the doctor do not disclose health information. Even when the doctor is a particular specialist or a psychologist, this information will not disclose protected information to unauthorized individuals. Advise the patient to call the office prior to the appointment if the patient has questions. This same guidance applies to postcard reminders.

B. *Myth—Prescription pickup:* Family members were afraid that only the patient would be able to pick up prescriptions at the local pharmacy.

   Proper response: Clearly a pharmacist is not to give prescriptions to just anyone who walks up to their counter. Patients may not be able to travel to a pharmacy or complete the paperwork required to receive their medications. Under HIPAA regulation, a family member or other individual may act on the patient's behalf to pick up medications, medical supplies, X-ray films, or other forms of PHI. The DHHS issued guidance on this topic in a press release on July 2001, stating "the rule allows a friend or relative to pick up a patient's prescription at the pharmacy." (HHS issues first guidance on new patient privacy protections, 2001). The health care provider is to use professional judgment and common practice to determine if releasing the medication, supplies, or other items is in the patient's best interest. Verification of identity is a reasonable precaution.

C. *Myth—Discussing patient information with family members:* A hospital or physician cannot share any information with the patient's family without the patient's written consent.

   Proper response: The Privacy Rule permits a health care provider to "disclose to a family member, other relative, or a close personal friend of the individual" medical information directly pertaining to the person's involvement with the patient, the patient's care, or for payment related to the patient's care. A health care professional may receive verbal consent from the patient when discussing patient care with the family member. If a family member is present and the patient does not object, the physician can infer that the patient is giving consent for the private discussion of health care. In situations where the patient is unable to give consent, the covered entity may determine whether the disclosure is in the patient's best interests. In each situation above, the permission verbally received, inferred, or the inability to authorize must be documented in the patient's medical record. Documentation is vital. Mantra for all health care workers: "Document, document, document." There cannot be too much documentation. It is better to have too much information than not enough.

D. *Myth—Refusal to sign the Notice of Privacy Practice:* A patient refuses to sign the acknowledgment of receipt of the Notice of Privacy Practices. Should the health care provider refuse to provide services?

   Proper response: The Privacy Rule requires that providers make a "good faith effort" to receive acknowledgment of the notice. The law does not give the provider the right to refuse services. Such offer of notice and the refusal to sign would be noted in the patient's record, but in no way does that deny them access to service or treatment. The signature of acknowledgment is not consent for treatment, nor is it authorization to release medical records, so it cannot be interpreted to mean more than the intended limited scope.

E. *Myth—Hospital patient list is eliminated:* Many people believed they could no longer find out the status of a friend who has been hospitalized. Some believed that the hospital directory listing was violation of the Privacy Rule.

   Proper response: The Privacy Rule permits hospitals to maintain a published listing of patients unless the patient has chosen to opt out. This option is to be made clear when the patient registers for admission. Information that may be disclosed is limited to their location in the facility, such as room and bed number, and their condition stated in general terms. Any inquirer must know the full name of the patient to receive the location and general condition. The choice to "opt-out" of the facility directory is mandated by HIPAA. Once this choice is made, it prohibits a facility from including that name on a *published* list of patients. Newspapers and other local media often are provided with list of patients in a hospital and discharge date. A facility has the option to write more stringent rules than HIPAA. In this case, it is no different than prior instances when some notable person has been hospitalized and rumor has circulated about the event. It may be an institutional policy to deny any knowledge of the individual being a patient due to their "Hollywood" status or political connections.

F. *Myth—Sharing of patient information between doctors:* Since consent and authorization were detailed in the NOPP, many providers assumed that nothing could be shared with a consulting physician without authorization.

   Proper response: The Privacy Rule permits providers who are involved in the direct treatment of a patient to share freely PHI without further authorization. Without this ability to discuss services or treatment of patients, the delivery of health care would be greatly impaired.

G. *Myth—Medical records are separate from other information on file:* Patients can only receive information that pertains directly to their health care. This can also include financial reports regarding payment or nonpayment of their account. Financial information, such as payments made by a health plan for a specific patient, belongs to the physician and does not come under the Privacy Rule for patient copy.

   Proper response: Patients can request a copy of their medical record. The patient may also request a *designated record set* of billing information. Records such as copies of a correspondence to a collection agency that the covered entity has on file may be designated and are considered legitimate requests under HIPAA law. The DHHS's Office for Civil Rights will help explain the patient's right to disclosure.

H. *Myth—Members of clergy are denied hospital information:* With the patient given the option to not reveal any information in hospital directory, many felt that clergy members would not be able to have a list of inpatients who may be members of their religious denomination.

   Proper response: Whether or not the patient has "opted-out" of the published directory lists, the patient may also be included on the denominational list of patients. Only clergy may then request a list of patients under their own denomination. The patient has the choice to opt out of this disclosure separately. Any policy more restrictive than this is an internal hospital policy rather than HIPAA law.

I. *Myth—PHI is disclosed in many new ways:* Patients received the NOPP. The list outlined when the HIPAA law allowed PHI to be disclosed and used. Many people felt this greatly increased the legal uses and disclosures of their PHI.

    Proper response: The DHHS mandates only two situations for disclosure: to the individual patient upon request and to the secretary of the DHHS for use in oversight investigations. Disclosures have long been required for purposes such as incidents of possible abuse, neglect, or domestic violence; national security; public health monitoring; and law enforcement. HIPAA does not conflict with or limit these permitted uses of disclosure.

J. *Myth—Patients will sue health care providers for noncompliance:* The fear of many providers is now that patients have written notice of when, where, and why PHI may be used, patients will feel any infraction is permission to begin a law suit.

    Proper response: The HIPAA Privacy Rule does not give people the right to sue a provider. Instead, if a person feels that the privacy of their information has been violated and has not received a satisfactory reply, a complaint may be filed with the regional office of the Office for Civil Rights where the alleged event took place. The OCR will investigate the complaint. If the health care provider is found to be in violation of HIPAA law or their own policy, the DHHS may impose civil penalties, and if flagrant violations are found, file criminal charges. However, the DHHS seeks to promote education and voluntary compliance and desires to work toward compliance rather than imposing penalties. It is very important for the provider to understand that violations are opportunities for education more than punishment.

    If the disclosure involves unauthorized disclosure of e-PHI, then the OHS, under CMS, is mandated to investigate complaints. Again, the DHHS seeks education and compliance unless there is flagrant violation, which is then turned over to the Department of Justice for criminal investigation.

K. *Myth—The press is prohibited from any public information from hospital personnel:* Members of the press will no longer be permitted any information about accident or crime victims from a hospital spokesperson.

    Proper response: Members of the press are to be treated just as any other person requesting information concerning a patient in the facility. Any patient may opt-out of disclosing their name on the published facility directory. Whether or not patients allow their name in a directory, they certainly do not want the provider's personnel talking to the press about their status. The location and general condition can be released to any individual asking for patient by full name unless an anonymity agreement is in place with the patient or their representative. If a state law restricts the hospital further, the state law takes precedence. Individual provider policy may be even more restrictive. Once a reporter legally receives patient information, the HIPAA law does not restrict the press in how they choose to convey the information given.

L. *Myth—Faxing of health information is now prohibited:* Fax machines have been widely used to send health information between providers. With the HIPAA Privacy Rule, the possible disclosure of PHI to unauthorized persons is punishable by law. Many facilities refuse to send any information by means of the fax machine.

Proper response: Fax machines have truly made life a lot easier to send and receive information quickly. With that ease comes some very large risks of improper disclosure. The machine must be in a secure location away from unauthorized access. An audit trail or record must be kept to document that information was sent to the proper location. This record is to be kept for six years. A cover sheet is necessary with disclaimers that this fax is intended for the designated person only. The best protection is to call the receiving party, send the fax information, and follow-up with another phone call to confirm receipt of information. Do not forget to log the confirmation.

Proper response when information is misdirected: If faxed health information is sent to the wrong phone number, immediate response is the best choice. Call the party that received the information and retrieve it if possible. If not retrievable, advise them to shred the papers immediately. Then make a notation in the patient's record of the error and what was done to remedy it. Notification of the patient should not be necessary unless sensitive medical information was disclosed without knowledge of who received the information.

M. *Myth—Patient access to records from another physician or health care facility not created by the facility:* An office requested and received reports from a referring doctor to assist with the treatment of a patient. That patient asks for a copy of his medical record. Can this facility include any information received from another doctor? Must the patient request the copy from the originating doctor?

Proper response: Once an office receives PHI and includes it with their files, it becomes part of the medical record set of documents.

These are to be included when a copy is requested. To claim that information from another source does not exist or that it is not part of the patient file denies that treatment and services were influenced by the information contained in the file.

SUMMARY

The DHHS has been instructed to provide national identifiers for each of the individuals and organizations that are named on a typical health insurance claim form. This list includes employers, physicians, health plans, and patients. Adoption of the patient identifier is not planned at the time of this writing due to public concerns. The other identifiers are being published currently. The employer identifier came first—the employer identification number (EIN) issued by the Internal Revenue Service; next, the physician identifier is the national provider identifier (NPI). The identifier for health plans is being developed. The Title II HIPAA ruling called Administrative Simplification is the first nationwide legislation to reform the health care industry. Standardization makes it a lot easier for individual covered entities to communicate with each other since it does away with unique qualifications previously demanded by particular health plans.

HIPAA was written to cover four areas.

1. *Ensure privacy* of individual health care information.

2. Enable employees to *continue health coverage* when moving to another job.

3. *Standardize electronic claims* transactions and related requests.

4. Keep all *health information secure* from adverse events or unauthorized access.

Patients who find their protected health information has been compromised are to file a compliant with the Office for Civil Rights. Other complaints involving security issues are submitted to the CMS and its Office for HIPAA Standards. The Department of Justice has decided a few criminal cases, and plaintiffs have been sentenced to jail times due to a combination of HIPAA violations and other violations of law.

Health care professionals need to be aware of possible medical identity theft. With new rulings come misconceptions about just how these rules are implemented. In all cases, the goal of HIPAA is to make reasonable changes so health care is improved and reimbursed in a more efficient manner.

REVIEW QUESTIONS

1. What four categories of identifiers has the HIPAA law mandated?

2. What transactions use the employer identification number (EIN)?

3. Why is it important that NPI not have "intelligence"?

4. Discuss objections to patient identifiers.

5. What advantages come with electronic access to medical records through a unique patient identification system? What are the disadvantages?

6. List two ways that unique health identifiers for patients would help physicians treat patients.

7. A patient is recovering after a minor surgical procedure. After recovery, the patient waits to receive final discharge instructions. If the patient's relative or friend is present too, instead of requesting to speak alone with the patient, is it permissible to say "I'd like to talk about discharge instructions with your relative present because it is often best to have another pair of ears to hear this information." Does this request cover the need for authorization to disclosure PHI?

8. A patient accounts worker calling to ask a patient questions concerning bill payment leaves a voice mail message on the patient's phone stating the doctor's office and phone number, and explains that payment is due in full within three business days. Is this acceptable information to leave on voice mail? If not, what would be a better message?

9. A patient is referred to a collection agency for failure to pay a bill or copayment. The patient requests a copy of the letter from the physician's office, but the office refused. Is this refusal in compliance with the Privacy Ruling since a letter to a collection agency is not part of the medical care or treatment of the patient?

10. Refer to a recent encounter with health care: How might someone be able to obtain medical services using another's identity? What safeguards were in place to prevent this type of theft from occurring?

11. Discuss how HIPAA Rule has already changed the delivery of health care. Note the advantages to the health care provider. Also note the disadvantages or roadblocks health care providers face with compliance.

REFERENCES

Davidson, K. E. & Holtz, D. L. (1998, October). Do unique identifiers violate patient privacy? *Physician's News Digest*, 11-12, p.8.

Electronic Transactions and Code Sets: An Overview, HIPAA Information Series. Volume 1 Paper 4, page 8. (May 2003). Retrieved from http://www.cms.gov.

Fact Sheet, Administrative Simplification Under HIPAA: National Standards for Transactions, Security and Privacy. (March 3, 2003). Department of Health and Human Services. Retrieved September 12, 2003, from http://www.hhs.gov/news/press/2002pres/hipaa.html

Health Insurance Reform: Standard Unique Employer Identifier, 45 C.F.R. Parts 160 and 162, 38,016 (May 30, 2002).

HHS issues first guidance on new patient privacy protections, HHS Press Office, Friday, July 6, 2001 retrieved from http://www.hhs.gov/news/press/2001pres/20010706a.html

HIPAA Administrative Simplification: Standard Unique Health Identifier for Health Care Providers, 69 Fed. Reg. 3,434–3,469. (Jan. 24, 2004) (to codify 45 C.F.R. Part 162).

Identifiers, Background papers. Retrieved February 23, 2004, from http://www.wedi.org/snip/public/articlesdetails~htm

Long, K. (2007, January). New IT buzzwords: 'medical identity theft'. *Healthcare IT News*, p. 1.

Mengers, P. (2004, May 2). The HIPAA effect II: Keeping it hush-hush. *Delco Times*. Retrieved January 19, 2007 from http://www.zwire.com/site/news.asp

Most AHIMA Survey Respondents Say HIPAA Uncovered "Problem Areas," *Report on Patient Privacy*. (May 2004). Atlantic Information Service, Inc., p. 3.

OIG launches audits of provider compliance with HIPAA security rule; Ga. hospital first. (2007. Feb. 26). *Report on Medicare Compliance*, Vol. 16, No. 8, p. 1.

Stein, R. Enforcement of HIPAA draws mixed reviews. *Fort Worth Star-Telegram (TX)* NewsBank, pg. A6. Retrieved January 19, 2007, from http://infoweb.newsbank.com

Unique Identifiers (including allowed uses). Retrieved html version February 25, 2004, from http://www.virtual.epm.br/material/healthcare/spanish/F_Refer3dd.pdf

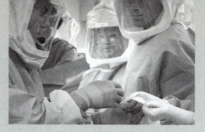

APPENDIX

HIPAA for Health Care Professionals

APPENDIX A: COVERED ENTITY CHARTS

Guidance on how to determine whether an organization or individual is a covered entity under the Administrative Simplification provisions of HIPAA

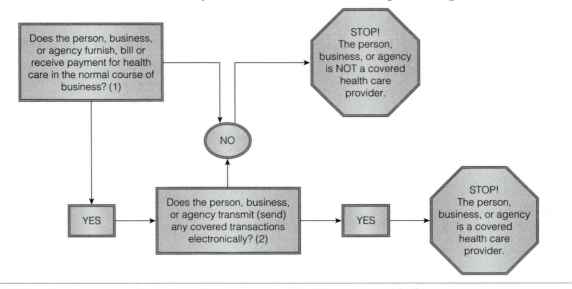

FORM 1: Is a person, business, or agency a covered health care provider?

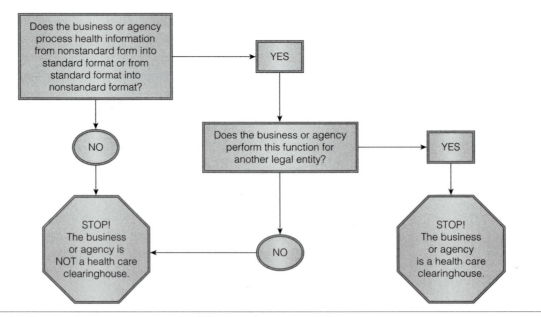

FORM 2: Is a business or agency a health care clearinghouse?

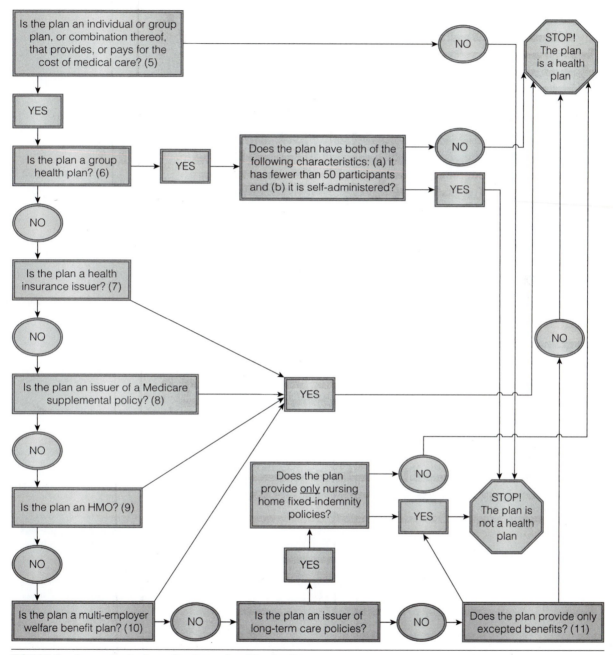

FORM 3:   Is a private benefit plan a health plan?

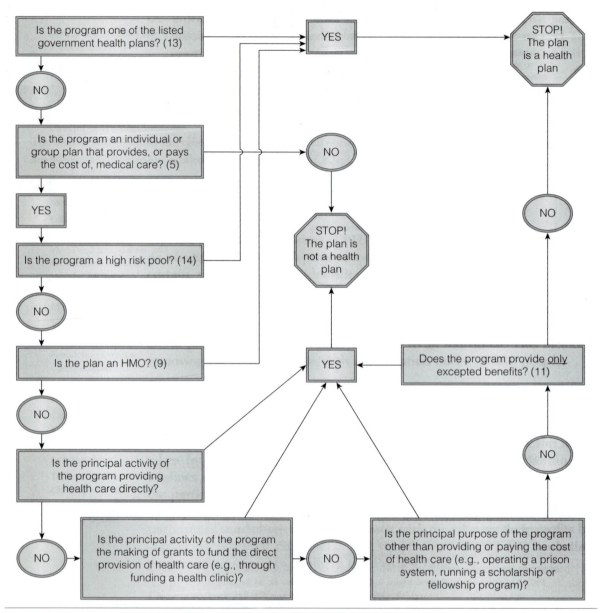

FORM 4: Is a government-funded program a health plan?

APPENDIX B: CMS REGIONAL OFFICES AND GOVERNMENT RESOURCES

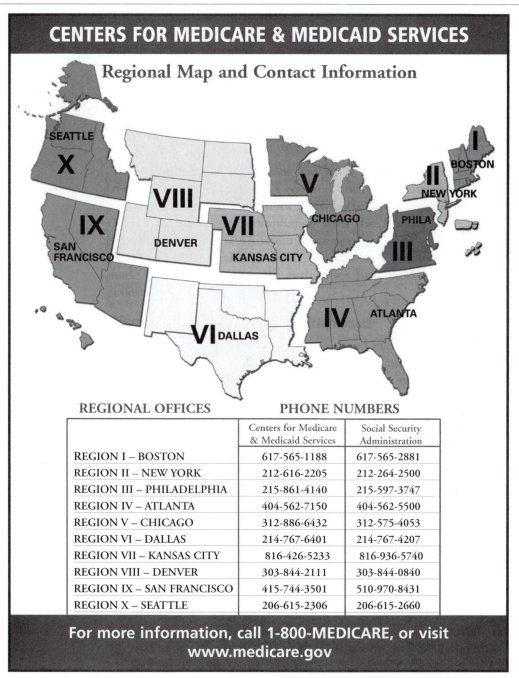

CENTERS FOR MEDICARE & MEDICAID SERVICES

Regional Map and Contact Information

REGIONAL OFFICES	PHONE NUMBERS	
	Centers for Medicare & Medicaid Services	Social Security Administration
REGION I – BOSTON	617-565-1188	617-565-2881
REGION II – NEW YORK	212-616-2205	212-264-2500
REGION III – PHILADELPHIA	215-861-4140	215-597-3747
REGION IV – ATLANTA	404-562-7150	404-562-5500
REGION V – CHICAGO	312-886-6432	312-575-4053
REGION VI – DALLAS	214-767-6401	214-767-4207
REGION VII – KANSAS CITY	816-426-5233	816-936-5740
REGION VIII – DENVER	303-844-2111	303-844-0840
REGION IX – SAN FRANCISCO	415-744-3501	510-970-8431
REGION X – SEATTLE	206-615-2306	206-615-2660

For more information, call 1-800-MEDICARE, or visit www.medicare.gov

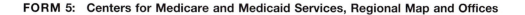

FORM 5:   Centers for Medicare and Medicaid Services, Regional Map and Offices

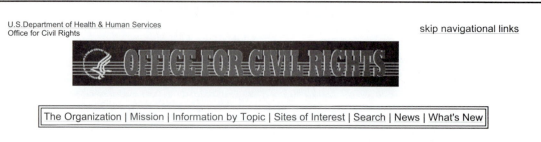

The Organization | Mission | Information by Topic | Sites of Interest | Search | News | What's New

Medical Privacy - National Standards to Protect the Privacy of Personal Health Information

SAMPLE BUSINESS ASSOCIATE CONTRACT PROVISIONS[1]
(Published in FR 67 No. 157 pg. 53182, 53264 (August 14, 2002))

Statement of Intent

The Department provides these sample business associate contract provisions in response to numerous requests for guidance. This is only sample language. These provisions are designed to help covered entities more easily comply with the business associate contract requirements of the Privacy Rule. However, use of these sample provisions is not required for compliance with the Privacy Rule. The language may be amended to more accurately reflect business arrangements between the covered entity and the business associate.

These or similar provisions may be incorporated into an agreement for the provision of services between the entities or they may be incorporated into a separate business associate agreement. These provisions only address concepts and requirements set forth in the Privacy Rule and alone are not sufficient to result in a binding contract under State law. They do not include many formalities and substantive provisions that are required or typically included in a valid contract. Reliance on this sample is not sufficient for compliance with State law and does not replace consultation with a lawyer or negotiations between the parties to the contract.

Furthermore, a covered entity may want to include other provisions that are related to the Privacy Rule but that are not required by the Privacy Rule. For example, a covered entity may want to add provisions in a business associate contract in order for the covered entity to be able to rely on the business associate to help the covered entity meet its obligations under the Privacy Rule. In addition, there may be permissible uses or disclosures by a business associate that are not specifically addressed in these sample provisions, for example having a business associate create a limited data set. These and other types of issues will need to be worked out between the parties.

Sample Business Associate Contract Provisions[2]

Definitions (alternative approaches)

Catch-all definition:

Terms used, but not otherwise defined, in this Agreement shall have the same meaning as those terms in the Privacy Rule.

FORM 6: Sample Business Associate Contract Provisions

Examples of specific definitions:

a. Business Associate. "Business Associate" shall mean [Insert Name of Business Associate].

b. Covered Entity. "Covered Entity" shall mean [Insert Name of Covered Entity].

c. Individual. "Individual" shall have the same meaning as the term "individual" in 45 CFR § 160.103 and shall include a person who qualifies as a personal representative in accordance with 45 CFR § 164.502(g).

d. Privacy Rule. "Privacy Rule" shall mean the Standards for Privacy of Individually Identifiable Health Information at 45 CFR Part 160 and Part 164, Subparts A and E.

e. Protected Health Information. "Protected Health Information" shall have the same meaning as the term "protected health information" in 45 CFR § 160.103, limited to the information created or received by Business Associate from or on behalf of Covered Entity.

f. Required By Law. "Required By Law" shall have the same meaning as the term "required by law" in 45 CFR § 164.103.

g. Secretary. "Secretary" shall mean the Secretary of the Department of Health and Human Services or his designee.

Obligations and Activities of Business Associate

a. Business Associate agrees to not use or disclose Protected Health Information other than as permitted or required by the Agreement or as Required By Law.

b. Business Associate agrees to use appropriate safeguards to prevent use or disclosure of the Protected Health Information other than as provided for by this Agreement.

c. Business Associate agrees to mitigate, to the extent practicable, any harmful effect that is known to Business Associate of a use or disclosure of Protected Health Information by Business Associate in violation of the requirements of this Agreement. [This provision may be included if it is appropriate for the Covered Entity to pass on its duty to mitigate damages to a Business Associate.]

d. Business Associate agrees to report to Covered Entity any use or disclosure of the Protected Health Information not provided for by this Agreement of which it becomes aware.

e. Business Associate agrees to ensure that any agent, including a subcontractor, to whom it provides Protected Health Information received from, or created or received by Business Associate on behalf of Covered Entity agrees to the same restrictions and conditions that apply through this Agreement to Business Associate with respect to such information.

(*continues*)

(continued)

f. Business Associate agrees to provide access, at the request of Covered Entity, and in the time and manner [Insert negotiated terms], to Protected Health Information in a Designated Record Set, to Covered Entity or, as directed by Covered Entity, to an Individual in order to meet the requirements under 45 CFR § 164.524. [Not necessary if business associate does not have protected health information in a designated record set.]

g. Business Associate agrees to make any amendment(s) to Protected Health Information in a Designated Record Set that the Covered Entity directs or agrees to pursuant to 45 CFR § 164.526 at the request of Covered Entity or an Individual, and in the time and manner [Insert negotiated terms]. [Not necessary if business associate does not have protected health information in a designated record set.]

h. Business Associate agrees to make internal practices, books, and records, including policies and procedures and Protected Health Information, relating to the use and disclosure of Protected Health Information received from, or created or received by Business Associate on behalf of, Covered Entity available [to the Covered Entity, or] to the Secretary, in a time and manner [Insert negotiated terms] or designated by the Secretary, for purposes of the Secretary determining Covered Entity's compliance with the Privacy Rule.

i. Business Associate agrees to document such disclosures of Protected Health Information and information related to such disclosures as would be required for Covered Entity to respond to a request by an Individual for an accounting of disclosures of Protected Health Information in accordance with 45 CFR § 164.528.

j. Business Associate agrees to provide to Covered Entity or an Individual, in time and manner [Insert negotiated terms], information collected in accordance with Section [Insert Section Number in Contract Where Provision (i) Appears] of this Agreement, to permit Covered Entity to respond to a request by an Individual for an accounting of disclosures of Protected Health Information in accordance with 45 CFR § 164.528.

Permitted Uses and Disclosures by Business Associate

General Use and Disclosure Provisions [(a) and (b) are alternative approaches]

a. Specify purposes:

Except as otherwise limited in this Agreement, Business Associate may use or disclose Protected Health Information on behalf of, or to provide services to, Covered Entity for the following purposes, if such use or disclosure of Protected Health Information would not violate the Privacy Rule if done by Covered Entity or the minimum necessary policies and procedures of the Covered Entity:
[List Purposes].

b. Refer to underlying services agreement:

Except as otherwise limited in this Agreement, Business Associate may use or disclose Protected Health Information to perform functions, activities, or services for, or on behalf of, Covered Entity as specified in [Insert Name of Services Agreement], provided that such use or disclosure would not violate the Privacy Rule if done by Covered Entity or the minimum necessary policies and procedures of the Covered Entity.

Specific Use and Disclosure Provisions [only necessary if parties wish to allow Business Associate to engage in such activities]

a. Except as otherwise limited in this Agreement, Business Associate may use Protected Health Information for the proper management and administration of the Business Associate or to carry out the legal responsibilities of the Business Associate.

b. Except as otherwise limited in this Agreement, Business Associate may disclose Protected Health Information for the proper management and administration of the Business Associate, provided that disclosures are Required By Law, or Business Associate obtains reasonable assurances from the person to whom the information is disclosed that it will remain confidential and used or further disclosed only as Required By Law or for the purpose for which it was disclosed to the person, and the person notifies the Business Associate of any instances of which it is aware in which the confidentiality of the information has been breached.

c. Except as otherwise limited in this Agreement, Business Associate may use Protected Health Information to provide Data Aggregation services to Covered Entity as permitted by 45 CFR § 164.504(e)(2)(i)(B).

d. Business Associate may use Protected Health Information to report violations of law to appropriate Federal and State authorities, consistent with § 164.502(j)(1).

Obligations of Covered Entity

Provisions for Covered Entity to Inform Business Associate of Privacy Practices and Restrictions [provisions dependent on business arrangement]

a. Covered Entity shall notify Business Associate of any limitation(s) in its notice of privacy practices of Covered Entity in accordance with 45 CFR § 164.520, to the extent that such limitation may affect Business Associate's use or disclosure of Protected Health Information.

b. Covered Entity shall notify Business Associate of any changes in, or revocation of, permission by Individual to use or disclose Protected Health Information, to the extent that such changes may affect Business Associate's use or disclosure of Protected Health Information.

c. Covered Entity shall notify Business Associate of any restriction to the use or disclosure of Protected Health Information that Covered Entity has agreed to in accordance with 45 CFR § 164.522, to the extent that such restriction may affect Business Associate's use or disclosure of Protected Health Information.

(continues)

(continued)

Permissible Requests by Covered Entity

Covered Entity shall not request Business Associate to use or disclose Protected Health Information in any manner that would not be permissible under the Privacy Rule if done by Covered Entity. [Include an exception if the Business Associate will use or disclose protected health information for, and the contract includes provisions for, data aggregation or management and administrative activities of Business Associate].

Term and Termination

a. Term. The Term of this Agreement shall be effective as of [Insert Effective Date], and shall terminate when all of the Protected Health Information provided by Covered Entity to Business Associate, or created or received by Business Associate on behalf of Covered Entity, is destroyed or returned to Covered Entity, or, if it is infeasible to return or destroy Protected Health Information, protections are extended to such information, in accordance with the termination provisions in this Section. [Term may differ.]

b. Termination for Cause. Upon Covered Entity's knowledge of a material breach by Business Associate, Covered Entity shall either:

   1. Provide an opportunity for Business Associate to cure the breach or end the violation and terminate this Agreement [and the _____ Agreement/ sections _____ of the _____ Agreement] if Business Associate does not cure the breach or end the violation within the time specified by Covered Entity;

   2. Immediately terminate this Agreement [and the _____ Agreement/ sections _____ of the _____ Agreement] if Business Associate has breached a material term of this Agreement and cure is not possible; or

   3. If neither termination nor cure are feasible, Covered Entity shall report the violation to the Secretary.

   [Bracketed language in this provision may be necessary if there is an underlying services agreement. Also, opportunity to cure is permitted, but not required by the Privacy Rule.]

c. Effect of Termination.

   1. Except as provided in paragraph (2) of this section, upon termination of this Agreement, for any reason, Business Associate shall return or destroy all Protected Health Information received from Covered Entity, or created or received by Business Associate on behalf of Covered Entity. This provision shall apply to Protected Health Information that is in the possession of subcontractors or agents of Business Associate. Business Associate shall retain no copies of the Protected Health Information.

   2. In the event that Business Associate determines that returning or destroying the Protected Health Information is infeasible, Business Associate shall provide to Covered Entity notification of the conditions that make return or destruction

infeasible. Upon [Insert negotiated terms] that return or destruction of Protected Health Information is infeasible, Business Associate shall extend the protections of this Agreement to such Protected Health Information and limit further uses and disclosures of such Protected Health Information to those purposes that make the return or destruction infeasible, for so long as Business Associate maintains such Protected Health Information.

Miscellaneous

a. Regulatory References. A reference in this Agreement to a section in the Privacy Rule means the section as in effect or as amended.

b. Amendment. The Parties agree to take such action as is necessary to amend this Agreement from time to time as is necessary for Covered Entity to comply with the requirements of the Privacy Rule and the Health Insurance Portability and Accountability Act of 1996, Pub. L. No. 104-191.

c. Survival. The respective rights and obligations of Business Associate under Section [Insert Section Number Related to "Effect of Termination"] of this Agreement shall survive the termination of this Agreement.

d. Interpretation. Any ambiguity in this Agreement shall be resolved to permit Covered Entity to comply with the Privacy Rule.

[1] *This website version of Sample Business Associate Contract Provisions was revised June 12, 2006 to amend the regulatory cites to the following terms: "individual"; "protected health information"; and "required by law."*

[2] *Words or phrases contained in brackets are intended as either optional language or as instructions to the users of these sample provisions and are not intended to be included in the contractual provisions.*

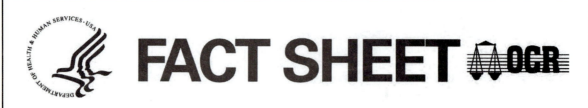

U.S. Department of Health and Human Services • Office for Civil Rights

HOW TO FILE A HEALTH INFORMATION PRIVACY COMPLAINT WITH THE OFFICE FOR CIVIL RIGHTS

If you believe that a person, agency or organization covered under the HIPAA Privacy Rule ("a covered entity") violated your (or someone else's) health information privacy rights or committed another violation of the Privacy Rule, you may file a complaint with the Office for Civil Rights (OCR). OCR has authority to receive and investigate complaints against covered entities related to the Privacy Rule. A covered entity is a health plan, health care clearinghouse, and any health care provider who conducts certain health care transactions electronically. For more information about the Privacy Rule, please look at our responses to Frequently Asked Questions (FAQs) and our Privacy Guidance. (See the web link near the bottom of this form.)

Complaints to the Office for Civil Rights must: (1) Be filed in writing, either on paper or electronically; (2) name the entity that is the subject of the complaint and describe the acts or omissions believed to be in violation of the applicable requirements of the Privacy Rule; and (3) be filed within 180 days of when you knew that the act or omission complained of occurred. OCR may extend the 180-day period if you can show "good cause." Any alleged violation must have occurred on or after April 14, 2003 (on or after April 14, 2004 for small health plans), for OCR to have authority to investigate.

Anyone can file written complaints with OCR by mail, fax, or email. If you need help filing a complaint or have a question about the complaint form, please call this OCR toll free number: 1-800-368-1019. OCR has ten regional offices, and each regional office covers certain states. You should send your complaint to the appropriate OCR Regional Office, based on the region where the alleged violation took place. Use the OCR Regions list at the end of this Fact Sheet, or you can look at the regional office map to help you determine where to send your complaint. Complaints should be sent to the attention off the appropriate OCR Regional Manager.

You can submit your complaint in any written format. We recommend that you use the OCR Health Information Privacy Complaint Form which can be found on our web site or at an OCR Regional office. If you prefer, you may submit a written complaint in your own format. Be sure to include the following information in your *written* complaint:

Your name, full address, home and work telephone numbers, email address.

If you are filing a complaint on someone's behalf, also provide the name of the person on whose behalf you are filing.

Name, full address and phone of the person, agency or organization you believe violated your (or someone else's) health information privacy rights or committed another violation of the Privacy Rule.

Briefly describe what happened. How, why, and when do believe your (or someone else's) health information privacy rights were violated, or the Privacy Rule otherwise was violated?

FORM 7:   How to File a Health Information Privacy Complaint with the Office for Civil Rights

Any other relevant information.

Please sign your name and date your letter.

The following information is optional:

Do you need special accommodations for us to communicate with you about this complaint?

If we cannot reach you directly, is there someone else we can contact to help us reach you?

Have you filed your complaint somewhere else?

The Privacy Rule, developed under authority of the Health Insurance Portability and Accountability Act of 1996 (HIPAA), prohibits the alleged violating party from taking retaliatory action against anyone for filing a complaint with the Office for Civil Rights. You should notify OCR immediately in the event of any retaliatory action. *To submit a complaint with OCR, please use one of the following methods.* If you mail or fax the complaint, be sure to follow the instructions above for determining the correct regional office.

Option 1: Open and print out the Health Information Privacy Complaint Form in PDF format (you will need Adobe Reader software) and fill it out. Return the completed complaint to the appropriate OCR Regional Office by mail or fax.

Option 2: Download the Health Information Privacy Complaint Form in Microsoft Word format to your own computer, fill out and save the form using Microsoft Word. Use the Tab and Shift/Tab on your keyboard to move from field to field in the form. Then, you can either: (a) print the completed form and mail or fax it to the appropriate OCR Regional Office; or (b) email the form to OCR at OCRComplaint@hhs.gov.

Option 3: If you choose not to use the OCR-provided Health Information Privacy Complaint Form (although we recommend that you do), please provide the information specified above and either: (a) send a letter or fax to the appropriate OCR Regional Office; or (b) send an email OCR at OCRComplaint@hhs.gov.

If you require an answer regarding a general health information privacy question, please view our Frequently Asked Questions (FAQs). If you still need assistance, you may call OCR (toll-free) at: 1-866-627-7748. You may also send an email to OCRPrivacy@hhs.gov with suggestions regarding future FAQs. Emails will not receive individual responses.

Website: http://www.hhs.gov/ocr/hipaa

(continues)

(continued)

Region I - CT, ME, MA, NH, RI, VT Office for Civil Rights U.S. Department of Health & Human Services JFK Federal Building - Room 1875 Boston, MA 02203 (617) 565-1340; (617) 565-1343 (TDD) (617) 565-3809 FAX	Region VI - AR, LA, NM, OK, TX Office for Civil Rights U.S. Department of Health & Human Services 1301 Young Street - Suite 1169 Dallas, TX 75202 (214) 767-4056; (214) 767-8940 (TDD) (214) 767-0432 FAX
Region II - NJ, NY, PR, VI Office for Civil Rights U.S. Department of Health & Human Services 26 Federal Plaza - Suite 3313 New York, NY 10278 (212) 264-3313; (212) 264-2355 (TDD) (212) 264-3039 FAX	Region VII - IA, KS, MO, NE Office for Civil Rights U.S. Department of Health & Human Services 601 East 12th Street - Room 248 Kansas City, MO 64106 (816) 426-7277; (816) 426-7065 (TDD) (816) 426-3686 FAX
Region III - DE, DC, MD, PA, VA, WV Office for Civil Rights U.S. Department of Health & Human Services 150 S. Independence Mall West - Suite 372 Philadelphia, PA 19106-3499 (215) 861-4441; (215) 861-4440 (TDD) (215) 861-4431 FAX	Region VIII - CO, MT, ND, SD, UT, WY Office for Civil Rights U.S. Department of Health & Human Services 1961 Stout Street - Room 1426 Denver, CO 80294 (303) 844-2024; (303) 844-3439 (TDD) (303) 844-2025 FAX
Region IV - AL, FL, GA, KY, MS, NC, SC, TN Office for Civil Rights U.S. Department of Health & Human Services 61 Forsyth Street, SW. - Suite 3B70 Atlanta, GA 30323 (404) 562-7886; (404) 331-2867 (TDD) (404) 562-7881 FAX	Region IX - AZ, CA, HI, NV, AS, GU, The U.S. Affiliated Pacific Island Jurisdictions Office for Civil Rights U.S. Department of Health & Human Services 90 7th Street, Suite 4-100 San Francisco, CA 94103 (415) 437-8310; (415) 437-8311 (TDD) (415) 437-8329 FAX
Region V - IL, IN, MI, MN, OH, WI Office for Civil Rights U.S. Department of Health & Human Services 233 N. Michigan Ave. - Suite 240 Chicago, IL 60601 (312) 886-2359; (312) 353-5693 (TDD) (312) 886-1807 FAX	Region X - AK, ID, OR, WA Office for Civil Rights U.S. Department of Health & Human Services 2201 Sixth Avenue - Mail Stop RX-11 Seattle, WA 98121 (206) 615-2290; (206) 615-2296 (TDD) (206) 615-2297 FAX

Saving, Retrieving or Emailing your data can only be done with the full version of the Adobe Acrobat or the Adobe Approval and not with the free Adobe Reader.

Form Approved: OMB No. 0990-0269.
See OMB Statement on Reverse.

DEPARTMENT OF HEALTH AND HUMAN SERVICES

OFFICE FOR CIVIL RIGHTS (OCR)

HEALTH INFORMATION PRIVACY COMPLAINT

If you have questions about this form, call OCR (toll-free) at:
1-800-368-1019 (any language) or 1-800-537-7697 (TDD)

YOUR FIRST NAME

YOUR LAST NAME

HOME PHONE

( )

WORK PHONE

( )

STREET ADDRESS

CITY

STATE

ZIP

E-MAIL ADDRESS *(If available)*

Are you filing this complaint for someone else? ☐ Yes ☐ No

If Yes, whose health information privacy rights do you believe were violated?

FIRST NAME

LAST NAME

Who (or what agency or organization, e.g., provider, health plan) do you believe violated your (or someone else's) health information privacy rights or committed another violation of the Privacy Rule?

PERSON / AGENCY / ORGANIZATION

STREET ADDRESS

CITY

STATE

ZIP

PHONE

( )

When do you believe that the violation of health information privacy rights occurred?

LIST DATE(S)

Describe briefly what happened. How and why do you believe your (or someone else's) health information privacy rights were violated, or the privacy rule otherwise was violated? Please be as specific as possible. *(Attach additional pages as needed)*

Please sign and date this complaint.

SIGNATURE

DATE

Filing a complaint with OCR is voluntary. However, without the information requested above, OCR may be unable to proceed with your complaint. We collect this information under authority of the Privacy Rule issued pursuant to the Health Insurance Portability and Accountability Act of 1996. We will use the information you provide to determine if we have jurisdiction and, if so, how we will process your complaint. Information submitted on this form is treated confidentially and is protected under the provisions of the Privacy Act of 1974. Names or other identifying information about individuals are disclosed when it is necessary for investigation of possible health information privacy violations, for internal systems operations, or for routine uses, which include disclosure of information outside the Department for purposes associated with health information privacy compliance and as permitted by law. It is illegal for a covered entity to intimidate, threaten, coerce, discriminate or retaliate against you for filing this complaint or for taking any other action to enforce your rights under the Privacy Rule. You are not required to use this form. You also may write a letter or submit a complaint electronically with the same information. To submit an electronic complaint, go to our web site at: **www.hhs.gov/ocr/privacyhowtofile.html** . To mail a complaint see reverse page for OCR Regional addresses.

HHS-670 (4/03) (FRONT)

FORM 8: Health Information Privacy Complaint form 2 pgs

(continues)

(continued)

(The remaining information on this form is optional. Failure to answer these voluntary questions will not affect OCR's decision to process your complaint.)

Do you need special accommodations for us to communicate with you about this complaint (check all that apply)?

☐ Braille ☐ Large Print ☐ Cassette tape ☐ Computer diskette ☐ Electronic mail ☐ TDD

☐ Sign language interpreter *(specify language)*:

☐ Foreign language interpreter *(specify language)*: ☐ Other:

If we cannot reach you directly, is there someone we can contact to help us reach you?

FIRST NAME

LAST NAME

HOME PHONE
( )

WORK PHONE
( )

STREET ADDRESS

CITY

STATE

ZIP

E-MAIL ADDRESS *(If available)*

Have you filed your complaint anywhere else? If so, please provide the following. (Attach additional pages as needed.)
PERSON / AGENCY / ORGANIZATION / COURT NAME(S)

DATE(S) FILED

CASE NUMBER(S) *(If known)*

To help us better serve the public, please provide the following information for the person you believe had their health information privacy rights violated (you or the person on whose behalf you are filing).

ETHNICITY *(select one)*   RACE *(select one or more)*

☐ Hispanic or Latino   ☐ American Indian or Alaska Native   ☐ Asian   ☐ Native Hawaiian or Other Pacific Islander

☐ Not Hispanic or Latino   ☐ Black or African American   ☐ White   ☐ Other *(specify)*:

PRIMARY LANGUAGE SPOKEN *(if other then English)*   HOW DID YOU LEARN ABOUT THE OFFICE FOR CIVIL RIGHTS?

To mail a complaint, please type or print, and return completed complaint to the OCR Regional Address based on the region where the alledged violation took place.

Region I - CT, ME, MA, NH, RI, VT
Office for Civil Rights
Department of Health & Human Services
JFK Federal Building - Room 1875
Boston, MA 02203
(617) 565-1340; (617) 565-1343 (TDD)
(617) 565-3809 FAX

Region V - IL, IN, MI, MN, OH, WI
Office for Civil Rights
Department of Health & Human Services
233 N. Michigan Ave. - Suite 240
Chicago, IL 60601
(312) 886-2359; (312) 353-5693 (TDD)
(312) 886-1807 FAX

Region IX - AZ, CA, HI, NV, AS, GU, The U.S. Affiliated Pacific Island Jurisdictions
Office for Civil Rights
Department of Health & Human Services
90 7th Street, Suite 4-100
San Francisco, CA 94103
(415) 437-8310; (415) 437-8311 (TDD)
(415) 437-8329 FAX

Region II - NJ, NY, PR, VI
Office for Civil Rights
Department of Health & Human Services
26 Federal Plaza - Suite 3313
New York, NY 10278
(212) 264-3313; (212) 264-2355 (TDD)
(212) 264-3039 FAX

Region VI - AR, LA, NM, OK, TX
Office for Civil Rights
Department of Health & Human Services
1301 Young Street - Suite 1169
Dallas, TX 75202
(214) 767-4056; (214) 767-8940 (TDD)
(214) 767-0432 FAX

Region X - AK, ID, OR, WA
Office for Civil Rights
Department of Health & Human Services
2201 Sixth Avenue - Mail Stop RX-11
Seattle, WA 98121
(206) 615-2290; (206) 615-2296 (TDD)
(206) 615-2297 FAX

Region III - DE, DC, MD, PA, VA, WV
Office for Civil Rights
Department of Health & Human Services
150 S. Independence Mall West - Suite 372
Philadelphia, PA 19106-3499
(215) 861-4441; (215) 861-4440 (TDD)
(215) 861-4431 FAX

Region VII - IA, KS, MO, NE
Office for Civil Rights
Department of Health & Human Services
601 East 12th Street - Room 248
Kansas City, MO 64106
(816) 426-7277; (816) 426-7065 (TDD)
(816) 426-3686 FAX

Region IV - AL, FL, GA, KY, MS, NC, SC, TN
Office for Civil Rights
Department of Health & Human Services
61 Forsyth Street, SW. - Suite 3B70
Atlanta, GA 30323
(404) 562-7886; (404) 331-2867 (TDD)
(404) 562-7881 FAX

Region VIII - CO, MT, ND, SD, UT, WY
Office for Civil Rights
Department of Health & Human Services
1961 Stout Street - Room 1426
Denver, CO 80294
(303) 844-2024; (303) 844-3439 (TDD)
(303) 844-2025 FAX

Burden Statement
Public reporting burden for the collection of information on this complaint form is estimated to average 45 minutes per response, including the time for reviewing instructions, gathering the data needed and entering and reviewing the information on the completed complaint form. An agency may not conduct or sponsor, and a person is not required to respond to, a collection of information unless it displays a valid control number. Send comments regarding this burden estimate or any other aspect of this collection of information, including suggestions for reducing this burden, to: HHS/OS Reports Clearance Officer, Office of Information Resources Management, 200 Independence Ave. S.W., Room 531H, Washington, D.C. 20201.

HHS-670 (4/03) (BACK)

APPENDIX C: HIPAA NON-PRIVACY COMPLAINT FORM

Form Approved: OMB # 0938-0948

CMS
CENTERS for MEDICARE & MEDICAID SERVICES

Centers for Medicare & Medicaid Services (CMS)
Office of E-Health Standards and Services (OESS)
HIPAA Non-Privacy Complaint Form

IMPORTANT: This form cannot be used for HIPAA Privacy complaints. Please direct privacy complaints to the Office for Civil Rights at 1-800-368-1019 or visit their website: **www.hhs.gov/ocr/hipaa**

If you have general questions about the HIPAA Regulations visit our website at: www.cms.hhs.gov

Please provide your contact information: (All fields required.)

YOUR NAME (First and Last)		ORGANIZATION NAME	
STREET ADDRESS		TELEPHONE NUMBER	
CITY/TOWN	COUNTY	STATE	ZIP

Who (or what agency/organization, e.g. health care clearinghouse, health plan, or covered health care provider) are you filing this complaint against? (All fields required.)

ORGANIZATION NAME		CONTACT NAME	
STREET ADDRESS		TELEPHONE NUMBER	
CITY/TOWN	COUNTY	STATE	ZIP

When did this alleged violation occur? mm/dd/yyyy (Required field.)

Identify the HIPAA Non-Privacy complaint category? (Required field.) Select one regulatory category listed below per complaint submission. Complete this form again to file a complaint for another category listed below.

☐ Transactions and Code Sets	☐ Unique Identifiers	☐ Security Standards

Describe, in detail, the alleged violation. (Required field.) You may attach additional pages as needed. Please enclose copies of any additional documents (e.g. companion guide, security risk assessment) that may help OESS resolve your complaint.

Please Print or Type.

Please sign and date this complaint. (Required field.)
SIGNATURE: DATE:

Filing a complaint with CMS is voluntary. However, without the information requested on the complaint form, CMS may be unable to proceed with a complaint. CMS collects this information under authority of 68 FR 60694 (October 23, 2003) issued pursuant to the HIPAA. CMS will use the information provided to determine if CMS has jurisdiction and, if so, how CMS will process the complaint. Information submitted on the complaint form is treated confidentially and is protected under the provisions of the Privacy Act of 1974. Names or other identifying information about individuals are disclosed only when it is necessary for investigation of possible HIPAA A.S. Non-Privacy violations, for internal systems operations, or for routine uses, which include disclosure of information outside the Department for purposes associated with HIPAA A.S. Non-Privacy compliance and as permitted by law. To submit an electronic complaint, go to our web site at: http://htct.hhs.gov

1

FORM 9: HIPAA Non-Privacy Compliant Form 3 pgs

Form Approved: OMB # 0938-0948

Centers for Medicare & Medicaid Services (CMS)

Office of E-Health Standards and Services (OESS)

HIPAA Non-Privacy Complaint Form

IMPORTANT: The information requested in the remainder of this form is optional. However, any additional information you provide will assist OESS in the enforcement process.

OPTIONAL INFORMATION

Have you filed this complaint with another agency? If so, please provide us with the following:

Agency Name:	Agency Contact Person:
Date the Complaint was Filed:	Contact Number:
Complaint Identification Number:	

Please provide OESS with more detail about this complaint.

1. **Please describe yourself.**
   - ❑ Health Plan
   - ❑ Covered Health Care Provider (*See examples on the right*)
   - ❑ Health Care Clearinghouse
   - ❑ Patient or representative of the patient
   - ❑ Other:_____

2. **Who are you filing this complaint against?**
   - ❑ Health Plan
   - ❑ Covered Health Care Provider (*See examples on the right*)
   - ❑ Health Care Clearinghouse

3. **Have you attempted to resolve the dispute?**
   - ❑ YES
   - ❑ NO

Examples of Covered Health Care Providers:
Ambulance Service
Comprehensive Outpatient Rehabilitation Facility
Durable Medical Equipment Service
Home Health Agency
Hospice Program
Hospital / Critical Access Hospital
Non-Physician Practitioners
Outpatient Physical or Occupational Therapy
Physician
Rural Health Clinics and Federally Qualified Health Centers
Skilled Nursing Facility

For a Transactions and Code Sets Complaint (Check the appropriate box.)

❑ **Non-Compliant Transaction Received** - You received a non-compliant HIPAA transaction from a covered entity.

❑ **Compliant Transaction Sent and Rejected** - A covered entity rejected your compliant HIPAA transaction.

❑ **Invalid Companion Guide** - A covered entity that you send data to or receive data from requires uses of a non-compliant companion guide. For example, a companion guide must not specify additional fields beyond those specified by HIPAA.

❑ **Code Set Received or Sent and Rejected:** - Either or both of these examples may apply: (1) A covered entity sent you a non-compliant HIPAA code within an electronic transaction. (2) A covered entity rejected a compliant HIPAA code that you sent within an electronic transaction.

❑ **Other** - You have another type of complaint against a covered entity.

Disclosure Statement: According to the Paperwork Reduction Act of 1995, no persons are required to respond to a collection of information unless it displays a valid OMB control number. The valid OMB control number for this information collection is **0938-0948**. The time required to complete this information collection is estimated to average **1 hour per** response, including the time to review instructions, search existing data resources, gather the data needed, and complete and review the information collection. If you have comments, concerning the accuracy of the time estimate(s) or suggestions for improving this form, please write to: CMS, 7500 Security Boulevard, Attn: PRA Reports Clearance Officer, Baltimore, Maryland 21244-1850.

Form Approved: OMB # 0938-0948

Centers for Medicare & Medicaid Services (CMS)
Office of E-Health Standards and Services (OESS)
HIPAA Non-Privacy Complaint Form

IMPORTANT: The information requested in the remainder of this form is optional. However, any additional information you provide will assist OESS in the enforcement process.

OPTIONAL INFORMATION

For a Transactions and Code Sets Complaint (Check the appropriate box.)

1. **Check the appropriate transaction(s) discussed in your complaint. Note: If your complaint involves a transaction(s) that is not listed, you may not have a valid transaction complaint.**

❑ 270 Eligibility, Coverage or Benefit Inquiry	❑ 837 Health Care Claim: Dental	❑ 835 Health Care Claim Payment/Advice
❑ 271 Eligibility, Coverage or Benefit Information	❑ 837 Health Care Claim – Professional	❑ 820 Payment Order/Remittance Advice
❑ 276 Health Care Claim Status Request	❑ 837 Health Care Claim: Institutional	❑ 278 Health Care Services Review - Request for Review
❑ 277 Health Care Claim Status Notification	❑ 834 Benefit Enrollment and Maintenance	❑ 278 Health Care Services Review - Response to Request for Review
❑ NCPDP Retail Pharmacy Transactions	❑ I don't know	

2. **Check the appropriate code set(s) discussed in your complaint.**

❑ International Classification of Diseases, 9th Edition, Clinical Modification (ICD-9-CM)	❑ Healthcare Common Procedure Coding System (HCPCS)
❑ Common Procedure Terminology (CPT)	❑ National Drug Code (NDC)
❑ Codes on Dental Procedures and Nomenclature - Current Dental Terminology (CDT)	❑ Other:_____

For a Security Complaint (Check the appropriate box.)

Do you believe that personal health information was wrongfully shared or disclosed, or that the action you are complaining about otherwise violated the health information Privacy Rule?

❑ YES

❑ NO

Mail completed forms to:	**Centers for Medicare & Medicaid Services**
	HIPAA Enforcement Activities
	P.O. Box 8030
	Baltimore, Maryland 21244-8030

Disclosure Statement: According to the Paperwork Reduction Act of 1995, no persons are required to respond to a collection of information unless it displays a valid OMB control number. The valid OMB control number for this information collection is **0938-0948**. The time required to complete this information collection is estimated to average **1 hour per** response, including the time to review instructions, search existing data resources, gather the data needed, and complete and review the information collection. If you have comments concerning the accuracy of the time estimate(s) or suggestions for improving this form, please write to: CMS, 7500 Security Boulevard, Attn: PRA Reports Clearance Officer, Baltimore, Maryland 21244-1850.

APPENDIX D: SECURITY STANDARDS MATRIX

5 Security Standards: Organizational, Policies and Procedures and Documentation Requirements

Security Standards Matrix (Appendix A of the Security Rule)

ADMINISTRATIVE SAFEGUARDS			
Standards	**Sections**	**Implementation Specifications** (R)= Required, (A)=Addressable	
Security Management Process	§ 164.308(a)(1)	Risk Analysis	(R)
		Risk Management	(R)
		Sanction Policy	(R)
		Information System Activity Review	(R)
Assigned Security Responsibility	§ 164.308(a)(2)		
Workforce Security	§ 164.308(a)(3)	Authorization and/or Supervision	(A)
		Workforce Clearance Procedure	(A)
		Termination Procedures	(A)
Information Access Management	§ 164.308(a)(4)	Isolating Health Care Clearinghouse Functions	(R)
		Access Authorization	(A)
		Access Establishment and Modification	(A)
Security Awareness and Training	§ 164.308(a)(5)	Security Reminders	(A)
		Protection from Malicious Software	(A)
		Log-in Monitoring	(A)
		Password Management	(A)
Security Incident Procedures	§ 164.308(a)(6)	Response and Reporting	(R)
Contingency Plan	§ 164.308(a)(7)	Data Backup Plan	(R)
		Disaster Recovery Plan	(R)
		Emergency Mode Operation Plan	(R)
		Testing and Revision Procedures	(A)
		Applications and Data Criticality Analysis	(A)
Evaluation	§ 164.308(a)(8)		
Business Associate Contracts and Other Arrangements	§ 164.308(b)(1)	Written Contract or Other Arrangement	(R)

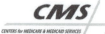

FORM 10:   Security Standards Matrix

5 Security Standards: Organizational, Policies and Procedures and Documentation Requirements

PHYSICAL SAFEGUARDS			
Standards	**Sections**	**Implementation Specifications** **(R)= Required, (A)=Addressable**	
Facility Access Controls	§ 164.310(a)(1)	Contingency Operations	**(A)**
		Facility Security Plan	**(A)**
		Access Control and Validation Procedures	**(A)**
		Maintenance Records	**(A)**
Workstation Use	§ 164.310(b)		
Workstation Security	§ 164.310(c)		
Device and Media Controls	§ 164.310(d)(1)	Disposal	**(R)**
		Media Re-use	**(R)**
		Accountability	**(A)**
		Data Backup and Storage	**(A)**
TECHNICAL SAFEGUARDS			
Standards	**Sections**	**Implementation Specifications** **(R)= Required, (A)=Addressable**	
Access Control	§ 164.312(a)(1)	Unique User Identification	**(R)**
		Emergency Access Procedure	**(R)**
		Automatic Logoff	**(A)**
		Encryption and Decryption	**(A)**
Audit Controls	§ 164.312(b)		
Integrity	§ 164.312(c)(1)	Mechanism to Authenticate Electronic Protected Health Information	**(A)**
Person or Entity Authentication	§ 164.312(d)		
Transmission Security	§ 164.312(e)(1)	Integrity Controls	**(A)**
		Encryption	**(A)**
ORGANIZATIONAL REQUIREMENTS			
Standards	**Sections**	**Implementation Specifications** **(R)= Required, (A)=Addressable**	
Business associate contracts or other arrangements	§ 164.314(a)(1)	Business Associate Contracts	**(R)**
		Other Arrangements	**(R)**
Requirements for Group Health Plans	§ 164.314(b)(1)	Implementation Specifications	**(R)**

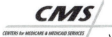

(continues)

(continued)

5 Security Standards: Organizational, Policies and Procedures and Documentation Requirements

POLICIES AND PROCEDURES AND DOCUMENTATION REQUIREMENTS			
Standards	**Sections**	**Implementation Specifications** **(R)= Required, (A)=Addressable**	
Policies and Procedures	§ 164.316(a)		
Documentation	§ 164.316(b)(1)	Time Limit	(R)
		Availability	(R)
		Updates	(R)

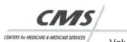

APPENDIX E: RESOURCES FOR HIPAA INFORMATION

Introduction to HIPAA—Chapter 1

1. Covered Entity Charts. Use to determine who is a covered entity as defined by CMS. http://www.cms.hhs.gov. Go to HIPAA General Information, Covered Entity Charts, pdf file.

2. Office for Civil Rights (OCR). DHHS department overseeing Privacy Rule enforcement. Responsible for overseeing compliance with the HIPAA Privacy Rules. http://www.hhs.gov/ocr. Search for HIPAA compliance.

Privacy Rule Resources—Chapter 2

3. Subscribe to HIPAA REGS listserv for notification via e-mail at http://www.cms.hhs.gov/hipaa/hipaa2/regulations/lsnotify.asp.

4. Centers for Medicare and Medicaid Services for HIPAA information. http://www.cms.gov/hipaa.

5. Government Printing Office for *Federal Register* documents and original source documents. http://www.access.gop.gov. Search for documents under the year, then date.

6. E-mail questions to the Centers for Medicare and Medicaid Services. http://askhipaa@cms.hhs.gov.

7. Centers for Medicare and Medicaid Services, HIPAA Hotline: 1-866-282-0659.

8. Department of Health and Human Services. This government Web site contains links to other government Web sites related to HIPAA Privacy, Transactions and Code Sets, and Security Rules. http://www.hhs.gov.

9. Health Privacy Project. The Health Privacy Project is dedicated to raising public awareness to the importance of ensuring health privacy so access and quality of health care is improved. http://www.healthprivacy.org.

10. HIPAA Advisory Site provided by Phoenix Health Systems, an information technology consulting and outsourcing company. There are many areas providing current HIPAA information and an e-mail subscription service. http://www.hipaadvisory.com.

Transactions and Code Sets Resources—Chapter 3

11. Centers for Disease Control and Prevention. http://www.cdc.gov.

12. World Health Organization. The organization that develops the International Classification of Diseases book. http://www.who.int.

13. American Health Information Management Association (AHIMA). http://www.ahima.org.

14. American Medical Association (AMA). The organization that maintains the Current Procedural Terminology coding system. http://www.ama.org.

15. Food and Drug Administration. http://www.fda.gov.

16. Government Web site for Designated Standard Maintenance Organizations (DSMO). http://www.hipaa-dsmo.org.

Names and Web Sites of Designated Standards Maintenance Organizations (DSMOs)—Chapter 3

17. Accredited Standards Committee X12. Develops transmission standards for business and industry transactions. http://www.x12.org.

18. Dental Content Committee of the American Dental Association. Develops dental procedures and Current Dental Terminology Version 4 codes. http://www.ada.org.

19. Health Level Seven. Develops transaction standards for claims attachments. http://www.hl7.org.

20. National Council for Prescription Drug Programs. Designated to maintain listing of drugs and biologics for retail pharmacy drug transactions. http://www.ncpdp.org.

21. National Uniform Billing Committee. Maintains standards for hospital billing form UB-92. http://www.nubc.org.

22. National Uniform Claim Committee. Maintains standards for HCFA-1500 physician services insurance claims. http://www.nucc.org.

Security Rule Resources—Chapter 4

23. Association for Electronic Health Care Transactions (AFECHT). http://www/afehct.org.

24. American Hospitals Association (AMA). http://www.hospitalconnect.com/DesktopServlet.

25. American Health Information Management Association (AHIMA). http://www.ahima.org.

26. American Health Lawyers Association (AHLA). http://www.ahla.org.

27. American Medical Informatics Association (AMIA). http://www.amia.org/resources/policy/f6.html.

28. Department of Health and Human Services (DHHS). http://aspe.os.dhhs.gov/admnsimp.

29. Department of Health and Human Services, Data Council. http://www.aspe.os.dhhs.gov/datacncl.

30. Strategic National Implementation Process, WEDI/SNIP Workgroup for Electronic Data Interchange (WEDI). Started the HIPAA project called Strategic National Implementation Process (SNIP). This group assists in the implementation of standards for administrative simplification mandated by HIPAA. http://www.wedi.org/snip.

31. Washington Publishing Company (WPC). The government source for implementation guides to all transactions. http://www.wpc-edi.com/HIPAA/HIPAA_40.asp.

32. National Infrastructure Protection Center (NIPC). Web site dealing with security issues for information systems. http://www.nipc.gov.

33. Submit an electronic version of nonprivacy complaint at http://htc/hhs.gov.

Identifier Rule Resources—Chapter 5

34. Office of E-Standards and Services (OESS). Coordinates implementation of comprehensive e-health strategy for CMS. Develops regulations, guidance materials and technical assistance on Administrative Simplification provisions of HIPAA. This office operates as a separate entity from CMS and related activities. http://www.cms.hhs.gov.

35. Office of HIPAA Standards (OHS). Authorized by CMS to implement HIPAA administrative simplification provisions. OESS serves as an access point to receive complaints from covered entities and others and directs the complaints to the proper office for investigation. The OHS receives the nonprivacy complaints regarding Security Rule, Transactions and Code Sets Rule, and Unique Identifier Rules. http://www.cms.hhs.gov/OHS.

36. Office of Inspector General (OIG). http://www.oig.hhs.gov. The area of DHHS that oversees enforcement of all rules and regulations issued by the Secretary of Health and Human Services. This office has delegated HIPAA enforcement to

    a. The Office for Civil Rights for enforcement of Privacy Rule violations

    b. CMS, which in turn organized the Office of HIPAA Standards for enforcement of Administrative Simplification violations dealing with the Transactions and Code Sets, Security, and Unique Identifier Rules. This office reports to the Office of E-Health Standards and Services with regard to complaints.

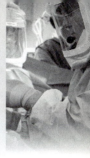

GLOSSARY

Access [4] ability or means necessary to read, write, modify, or communicate data and/or information or otherwise use any system resource

ADA [3] American Dental Association

Adjudication [3] final determination of the issues involving settlement of an insurance claim; also known as a claim settlement

Administrative safeguards [4] administrative actions, plus policies and procedures, 1) to manage the selection, development, implementation, and maintenance of security measures that protect electronic protected health information; and 2) to manage the conduct of the covered entity's workforce in relation to the protection of that information

AHIMA [2] American Health Information Management Association

Algorithm [4] step-by-step procedure for solving a problem or accomplishing some end, especially by a computer

AMA [3] American Medical Association

ANSI [3] American National Standards Institute

ASC X12 standard [3] Accredited Standards Committee–developed uniform standards (X12) for interindustry electronic exchange of business transactions by means of electronic data interchange (EDI).

ASET [4] Administrative Simplification Enforcement Tool; Web site where one may file a nonprivacy complaint concerning HIPAA security or the Transaction and Code Sets rule

ASTM [5] American Society for Testing and Materials

Audit trail [4] data collected during the use of electronic devices that includes the "who" (login ID), "what" (read-only, modify, delete, add, etc.), "where" (which device was accessed), and "when" (date/time stamp). This data may be used to facilitate a security audit.

Authentication [4] corroboration or confirmation that a person is the one claimed

Authorization [2] written permission by the patient or the patient's personal representative allowing the use or disclosure of specific protected health information for purposes other than treatment, payment, and health care operations

BA [1] business associate

Biologic [3] product used in the manufacture of medicine

Business associate (BA) [2] person or organization that performs or assists a function or activity on behalf of a covered entity, but is not part of the covered entity's workforce. Functions may involve the use or disclosure of individually identifiable health information, including claims processing; data analysis, processing, or administration; utilization review; quality assurance; billing; benefit management; practice management; and repricing. A business associate may be someone who provides legal, actuarial, accounting, consulting, accreditation, or financial services to or for a covered entity. A business associate can also be a covered entity in its own right.

CAT [2] computerized axial tomography

CHAMPVA [1] Civilian Health and Medical Program of the Veterans Administration

Check digit [5] digit that provides a means to check that a number is accurate. The usual algorithm sums the nine digits until a single digit is placed in the "ones" column as the check. If numbers are transposed or entered in error, the check digit will not match and an error will be spotted.

CLIA [1] Clinical Laboratory Improvement Amendments

CMS [1] Centers for Medicare and Medicaid Services

CMS-1500 [1] claim form used by physicians to bill health plans for their services

COB [3] Coordination of Benefits

COBRA [1] Consolidated Omnibus Budget Reconciliation Act of 1985

Code set [3] any set of codes used to encode data elements, such as tables of terms, medical concepts, medical diagnostic codes, or medical procedure codes. A code set includes the codes and the descriptors (words of description) of the codes.

Consent [2] permission granted by the patient or the patient's representative to use or disclose protected health information for purposes of treatment, payment, or health care operations

Contingency plan [4] policies and procedures for responding to an emergency or other occurrence that damages systems containing e-PHI. This is also called a "business continuity plan."

Covered entity [1] health plan, health care clearinghouse, or health care provider who transmits any health information in electronic form in connection with a transaction covered by HIPAA's Administrative Simplification provisions. If a provider uses another entity to conduct covered transactions in electronic form on its behalf, the health care provider is considered to be conducting the transaction in electronic form.

CPRI [5] Computer-based Patient Record Institute

CPT-4 [3] *Current Procedural Terminology*, 4th edition

CPU [4] central processing unit of a computer

Crossover claim [3] Medicare claim that Medicare transmits electronically to the secondary coverage health plan, usually but not always a Medicaid or Medigap plan.

DHHS [1] Department of Health and Human Services

De-identified health information [2] health information that does not identify or provide a reasonable basis to identify an individual

Designated record set [2] group of related data maintained by or for a covered entity that includes the medical records and billing records about individuals maintained by or for a covered health care provider; the enrollment, payment, claims adjudication, and case or medical management record systems maintained by or for a health plan; or information used, in whole or in part, by or for the covered entity to make decisions about individuals. Disclosure of medical information must define or designate the extent of the disclosure, e.g., the EKG tracing, or the complete medical records for an encounter covering specified dates, or the employment status of a subscriber to a health plan.

Diagnostic and Statistical Manual of Mental Disorders, 4th Edition, Text Revision (DSM-IV-TR) [3] reference book used by mental health providers to designate specific mental illnesses. This reference was not adopted as a standard code set by the DHHS under HIPAA law.

Disclosure of protected health information (PHI) [2] release, transfer, divulging of, or providing access to protected health information to an outside entity

DOJ [2] Department of Justice

EDI [1] electronic data interchange

EIN [5] employer identification number

Electronic data interchange (EDI) [3] computer-to-computer transmission of business information in a standard format using national standard communications protocols

E/M [3] evaluation and management services

Emancipated minor [2] person younger than eighteen (18) years of age who lives independently, is totally self-supporting, is married or divorced, is a parent even if not married, or is in the military, and possesses decision-making rights.

Employer identification number (EIN) [5] taxpayer identifying number of an individual or other entity assigned by the Internal Revenue Service as the taxpayer on documents as explained in the Internal Revenue Code.

EMR [3] electronic medical record

Encryption [4] use of an algorithmic process to transform data into a format in which there is a low probability of assigning meaning without use of a confidential process or key; transforming confidential plain text into cipher text to protect it. Once encrypted, data can be stored or transmitted over unsecured lines.

EOB [3] explanation of benefits

e-PHI [1] electronic protected health information

Etiology [3] all causes of a disease or abnormal condition

Explanation of Benefits (EOB) [3] written listing of services sent to the patient or guarantor by the health plan showing what the provider billed the health plan. The EOB includes the amount paid by the health plan for each procedure charged, the amount posted toward the deductible, if applicable, and the amount that may be the guarantor's responsibility pending a statement by the provider.

FAQ [5] frequently asked questions

Format [3] those data elements that provide or control the enveloping or hierarchical structure, or assist in identifying data content of a transaction

Group health plan [1] employee welfare benefit plan that provides health coverage in the form of medical care, including items and services paid for as medical care, to employees or their dependents directly or through insurance, reimbursement or otherwise, and that 1) has 50 or more participants, or 2) is administered by an entity other than the employer that established and maintains the plan. It may be sponsored by an employer or a union and includes private employer plans, Federal governmental plans, nonfederal governmental plans, and church plans. See 45 C.F.R. 160.103.

HCPCS [3] Health [Care Financing Administration] Common Procedure Coding System ("hick-picks"). A coding system maintained by Centers for Medicare and Medicaid Services (CMS) for nonphysician services like, but not limited to, such things as medical supplies, orthotic and prosthetic devices, and durable medical equipment.

Health care [1] care, services, or supplies related to the health of an individual. It includes, but is not limited to, the following: 1) preventive, diagnostic, rehabilitative, maintenance, or palliative care, and counseling, service, assessment, or procedures with respect to the physical or mental condition, or functional status, of an individual or that affects the structure or function of the body; and 2) sale or dispensing of a drug, device, equipment, or other item in accordance with a prescription. See 45 C.F.R. 160.103.

Health care clearinghouse [1] public or private entity that performs either of the following functions: 1) processing (or facilitating the processing of) information received from another entity in a nonstandard format or containing nonstandard data content into standard data elements or a standard transaction; or 2) receiving a standard transaction from another entity and processing (or facilitating the processing of) information into nonstandard format or nonstandard data content for the receiving entity. (Entities including, but not limited to, billing services, repricing companies, community health management information systems, or community health information systems, as well as "value-added" networks, if they perform these functions, are health care clearinghouses.)

Health care operations [2] certain administrative, financial, legal, and quality improvement activities of a covered entity that are necessary to run its business and to support the core functions of treatment and payment

Health care provider [1] provider of medical or other health services and any other person who furnishes, bills, or is paid for health care in the normal course of business

Health Insurance Portability and Accountability Act of 1996 (HIPAA) [1] federal law that allows persons to qualify immediately for comparable health insurance coverage when they change their employment relationships. Title II, subtitle F, of HIPAA gives DHHS the authority to mandate the use of standards for the electronic exchange of health care data; to specify what medical and administrative code sets should be used within those standards; to require the use of national identification systems for health care patients, providers, payers (or plans), and employers (or sponsors); and to specify the types of measures required to protect the security and privacy of personally identifiable health care information. Also known as the Kennedy-Kassebaum Bill, the Kassebaum-Kennedy Bill, K2, or Public Law 104-191.

Health maintenance organization (HMO) [1] federally qualified health maintenance organization, an organization recognized as a health maintenance organization under state law, or a similar organization regulated for solvency under state law in the same manner. See 45 C.F.R. 160.103. CMS definition: "A type of Medicare managed care plan where a group of doctors, hospitals, and other health care providers agree to give health care to Medicare beneficiaries for a set amount of money from Medicare every month. You usually must get your care from the providers in the plan."

Health plan [2] entity that assumes the risk of paying for some or all medical treatments, i.e., uninsured patient, self-insured employer, payer, or HMO, as outlined in their policy coverage. Examples of various plans are group health plan, health insurance issuer, health maintenance organization, Part A or Part B of Medicare, Medicaid program, Medicare supplemental policy, long-term care policy, employee welfare benefit plan, health care program for active military personnel, veterans health care program (CHAMPVA), Civilian Health and Medical Program of the Uniformed Services (CHAMPUS), Indian health service program, and Federal Employees Health Benefit Plan.

HEDIS [2] health plan employer data and information set

HIPAA [1] see Health Insurance Portability and Accountability Act of 1996

HIPAA officer [1] person responsible in each covered entity for keeping abreast of HIPAA rulings and in turn training and educating the rest of the workforce on how to comply with the rulings

HL7 [3] Health Level Seven, an organization responsible to develop electronic standards

HMO [3] health maintenance organization

ICD-9-CM [3] International Classification of Diseases, ninth revision, Clinical Modifications

IIHI [1] individually identifiable health information

Incidental disclosure [2] disclosure of individually identifiable health information (IIHI) as a result of or as "incident to" an otherwise permitted use or disclosure

Individually identifiable health information (IIHI) [1] any protected health information about an individual that can possibly identify that individual with the medical information included

Information system [4] interconnected set of information resources under the same direct management control that shares common functionality. A system normally includes hardware, software, information, data, applications, communications, and people.

Infrastructure [4] underlying foundation or basic framework (as of a system or organization), including hardwired and wireless networks, servers, routers, and other hardware and software, that directs information system commands and responses and transports and stores data.

Integrity [4] property (of data or information) of having not been altered or destroyed in an unauthorized manner

IRB [2] institutional review board

IRS [5] Internal Revenue Service

ISO [5] International Standards Organization

LAN [4] local area network

Limited data set [2] protected health information (PHI) that excludes the following direct identifiers of the individual or of relatives, employers, or household members of the individual: names, postal address information, telephone numbers, fax numbers, electronic mail addresses, social security numbers, medical record numbers, health plan beneficiary numbers, account numbers, certificate and license numbers, vehicle identifiers and serial numbers, license plate numbers, device identifiers and serial numbers, biometric identifiers, and full-face photographic images or comparable images.

Marketing [2] any communication about a product or service that encourages recipients to purchase or use the product or service unless the communication is 1) to describe a health-related product or service provided by or included in the plan of benefits of the covered entity; 2) for treatment of the individual; 3) for case management or care coordination for the individual or to recommend alternative treatments, therapies, health care providers, or settings of care to the individual.

MCO [3] managed care organization

Medical care [1] amounts paid for 1) diagnosis, cure, mitigation, treatment, or prevention of disease, or amounts paid for the purpose of affecting any structure or function of the body; 2) amounts paid for transportation, primarily for that essential to medical care referred to in 1); and 3) amounts paid for insurance covering medical care referred to in 1) and 2). See 42 U.S.C.300GG-91 (A)(2).

Medical identity theft [5] obtaining by theft or deception personal medical information, such as one's address, social security number, or health insurance information, for use in submitting false claims or seeking medical care or goods

Medical savings account (MSA) [1] tax-sheltered savings account similar to the individual retirement account, (IRA), but earmarked for medical expenses only. Deposits are 100 percent tax-deductible for the self-employed and can be easily withdrawn by check or debit card to pay routine medical bills with tax-free dollars.

Minimum necessary [2] When using or disclosing PHI or when requesting PHI from a covered entity, reasonable efforts must be made to limit PHI to only that which is necessary to accomplish the intended purposes of the use, disclosure, or request.

MRI [2] magnetic resonance imaging

MSA [1] medical savings accounts, legislation has expanded MSAs to include health savings accounts also.

NABP [5] National Association of Boards of Pharmacy

National provider identifier (NPI) [5] system for uniquely identifying all providers of health care services, supplies, and equipment. A term proposed by the secretary of HHS as the standard identifier for health care providers.

NDC [3] National Drug Code

Need to know [1] security principle stating that a user should have access only to the data he or she needs to perform a particular function

Nomenclature [3] designation; the act or process of naming

Nonrepudiation security [4] method by which the sender of data is provided with proof of delivery and the recipient is assured of the sender's identity so that neither can later deny having processed the data

NOPP [1] Notice of Privacy Practices

NPI [5] national provider identifier

NUBC [5] National Uniform Billing Committee

NUCC [5] National Uniform Claim Committee

OCR [2] Office for Civil Rights

OESS [3] Office of E-Health Standards and Services

Office for Civil Rights (OCR) [2] The Health and Human Services Department has authorized the OCR to investigate all complaints of violation of the Privacy Rule.

Office of E-Health Standards and Services (OESS) [3] This office develops and coordinates implementation of a comprehensive e-health strategy for CMS. The OESS develops regulations and guidance materials, and provides technical assistance on the Administrative Simplification provisions of HIPAA, including transactions, code sets, identifiers, and security. They also develop and implement the enforcement program for HIPAA's Administrative Simplification provisions. This office is not responsible for enforcement of the Privacy Rule; it is enforced by the Office for Civil Rights. This office is a separate entity and completely detached from CMS's Medicare and Medicaid programs.

Office of HIPAA Standards (OHS) [3] The secretary of DHHS created this office in 2002 to proactively support and oversee HIPAA transaction and code set standards (TCS) requirements, security requirements, and national identifier requirements. Further functions are to establish and operate enforcement processes related to HIPAA standards for Transactions and Code Sets Rule, the Security Rule and the Unique Identifier Rules.

OHS [3] Office of HIPAA Standards, under CMS

Opt-out [2] patient's decision that a health care facility may not publish his or her name, location, and general condition in a printed directory for distribution purposes

Orthotic [3] support or brace for weak or ineffective joints or muscles

OTC [3] over-the-counter

Password [4] confidential character string used in conjunction with a user ID to verify the identity of an individual attempting to gain access to a computer system

PCP [1] primary care physician

PDA [4] personal data assistant

PDP [1] prescription drug plan

Physical safeguards [4] physical measures, policies, and procedures to protect a covered entity's electronic information systems and related buildings and equipment from natural and environmental hazards and unauthorized intrusion

PIN [4] personal identification number

PPO [3] preferred provider organization

Privacy [1] an individual's claim to control the use and disclosure of personal information. This claim is backed by the societal value representing that claim.

Protected health information (PHI) [2] individually identifiable health information transmitted or maintained in any form or medium, which is held by a covered entity or its business associate, and that 1) identifies the individual or offers a reasonable basis for identification; 2) is created or received by a covered entity or an employer; 3) relates to a past, present, or future physical or mental condition, provision of health care, or payment for health care.

Protocol [3] set of conventions governing the treatment and especially the formatting of data in an electronic communications system; a code prescribing strict adherence to correct etiquette and precedents.

Provider taxonomy code [3] standard administrative code set for identifying the health care provider type and area of specialization of health care providers. This was replaced with NPI beginning in 2007.

Psychotherapy notes [2] notes recorded (in any medium) by a health care provider who is a mental health professional that document or analyze the contents of conversations during a private counseling session or a group, joint, or family counseling session and that are separated from the rest of the individual's medical record. Psychotherapy notes exclude medication prescription and monitoring, counseling session start and stop times, the modalities and frequencies of treatment furnished, results of clinical tests, and any summary of the following items: diagnosis, functional status, treatment plan, symptoms, prognosis, and progress to date.

Risk [4] impact and likelihood of an adverse event; possibility of harm or loss to any software, information, hardware, administrative, physical, communications, or personnel resource within an automated information system or activity

Risk analysis [4] process whereby cost-effective security control measures may be selected by balancing the cost of various security control measures against the losses that would be expected if these measures were not in place

Risk management [4] ongoing process that assesses the risk to electronic information resources and the information itself to determine adequate security for a system that will reduce the threats and vulnerabilities to protected health information to a minimal, acceptable amount

Security of electronic protected health information (e-PHI) [4] safeguards (administrative, technical, or physical) in an information system that protect it and its information against unauthorized disclosure and limit access to authorized users in accordance with an established policy

Security incident [4] attempted or successful unauthorized access, use, disclosure, modification, or destruction of information or interference with system operations in an information system

SSN [5] social security number

Subscriber [3] person whose name is listed in a health insurance policy

SUEI [5] standard unique employer identifier

Taxonomy codes [3] administrative codes to identify the provider type and specialization for all health care providers used in a HIPAA-covered transaction. The national provider identifier eliminates any means to identify specialty information about the provider.

TCS [1] transactions and code sets

Technical safeguards [4] technology and the policy and procedures for its use that protect electronic protected health information and control access to it

TIN [5] tax identification number

TPA [3] trading partner agreement

TPO [1] treatment, payment, or health care operation

Trading partner [3] external entity with whom business is conducted, i.e., a customer. This relationship can be formalized via a trading partner agreement. (Note: one that is a trading partner of an entity for some purposes may be a business associate of that same entity for other purposes.)

Trading partner agreement (TPA) [3] agreement related to the exchange of information in electronic transactions, whether the agreement is distinct or part of a larger agreement, between each party to the agreement. (For example, a trading partner agreement may specify, among other things, the duties and responsibilities of each party to the agreement in conducting a standard transaction.) This is *not* required by HIPAA.

Transaction [1] under HIPAA, signifies the exchange of electronic information between two parties to carry out financial or administrative activities related to health care using a specific standardized format. These are transactions for which the secretary of Health and Human Services has adopted standards; the standards are listed in 45 C.F.R. Part 162. If a health care provider uses another entity (such as a clearinghouse) to conduct covered transactions in electronic form on its behalf, the health care provider is considered to be conducting the transaction in electronic form.

Treatment [2] provision, coordination, or management of health care and related services for an individual by one or more health care providers or by a health care provider with a third party, including consultation between health care providers regarding a patient and referral of a patient from one health care provider to another

TRICARE [1] health coverage program for members and beneficiaries of uniformed services, formerly called CHAMPUS—Civilian Health and Medical Program for Uniformed Services

Use of protected health information (PHI) [2] sharing, employment, application, utilization, examination, or analysis of individually identifiable health information (IIHI) within an entity that maintains such information

UB-04 [3] Uniform Billing–2004; replaced hospital billing form UB-92

UHID [5] universal health identifier

UPIN [5] unique physician identification numbers

User [4] person or entity with authorized access

VPN [4] virtual private network

WEDI [5] Workgroup for Electronic Data Interchange

WHO [3] World Health Organization

Workforce [2] employees, volunteers, trainees, and other persons under the direct control of a covered entity, whether or not they are paid by the covered entity

Workstation [4] electronic computing device; for example, a laptop or desktop computer, or any other device that performs similar functions including the electronic media stored in its immediate environment

X12N [3] subcommittee of ASC/X12 that defines electronic data interchange (EDI) standards for the insurance industry

INDEX

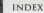